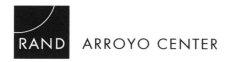

The Neurological Effects of Repeated Exposure to Military Occupational Blast

Implications for Prevention and Health

PROCEEDINGS, FINDINGS, AND EXPERT RECOMMENDATIONS
FROM THE SEVENTH ANNUAL DEPARTMENT OF DEFENSE
STATE-OF-THE-SCIENCE MEETING, 12–14 MARCH, 2018

Charles C. Engel, Emily Hoch, Molly Simmons

Editors

Prepared for the United States Army

Approved for public release; distribution unlimited

For more information on this publication, visit www.rand.org/t/CF380z1

Library of Congress Cataloging-in-Publication Data is available for this publication.
ISBN: 978-1-9774-0206-6

Published by the RAND Corporation, Santa Monica, Calif.

© Copyright 2019 RAND Corporation

RAND® is a registered trademark.

Cover photos (clockwise from top left): U.S. Army photo by Spec. Donald Williams;
U.S. Air Force photo by Staff Sgt. Evelyn Chavez; U.S. Marine Corps photo by Sgt. Mauricio Campino;
Department of Defense photo by Cpl. Tyler Main; U.S. Air Force photo; U.S. Army photo by Sgt. Michael Eaddy.

Support RAND
Make a tax-deductible charitable contribution at
www.rand.org/giving/contribute

www.rand.org

Preface

There has been growing concern over potential subconcussive neurological injury following repetitive low-level military occupational blast exposure (MOB). Examples include heavy weapons training and activities such as breaching. To address this issue, the Seventh Department of Defense (DoD) State-of-the-Science Meeting (SoSM) was held March 12–15, 2018, at the RAND Corporation's offices in Arlington, Virginia. These proceedings include background information on the meeting and its theme, summaries of a systematic RAND Arroyo Center literature review and meeting and poster presentations, and complete working group findings and expert panel conclusions and recommendations.

The SoSM expert panel recommended that DoD leaders (1) enforce DoD policies and standards related to low-level MOB; (2) develop high-quality research assessing the occurrence of repeated, low-level occupational blast injury; (3) plan and complete a large-scale population-based longitudinal study of military personnel with long follow-up to assess neurological and general health outcomes after repeated, low-level MOB exposure; (4) emphasize research on large animals, including nonhuman primates, as part of the department's animal research initiatives to improve the applicability of findings to humans; (5) complete studies that compare extant MOB exposure assessment tools, protective practices, and protective devices with improvement approaches to facilitate incremental gains in safety and outcomes; (6) catalogue, map, and make available to researchers, safety programs, and military end users unclassified weapon system–specific information and service member–specific load profiles for key military occupations, exposures, and contexts; and (7) increase opportunities for embedded scientists to study low-level MOB exposure among training units and in deployed contexts.

The meeting and these proceedings were sponsored by the Army Medical Research and Materiel Command.

The Project Unique Identification Code (PUIC) for the project that produced this document is RAN177782.

This research was conducted within RAND Arroyo Center's Personnel, Training, and Health Program. RAND Arroyo Center, part of the RAND Corporation, is a federally funded research and development center (FFRDC) sponsored by the United States Army.

RAND operates under a "Federal-Wide Assurance" (FWA00003425) and complies with the *Code of Federal Regulations for the Protection of Human Subjects Under United States Law* (45 CFR 46), also known as "the Common Rule," as well as with the implementation guidance set forth in DoD Instruction 3216.02. As applicable, this compliance includes reviews and approvals by RAND's Institutional Review Board (the Human Subjects Protection Committee) and by the U.S. Army. The views of participants are solely their own and do not represent the official policy or position of DoD or the U.S. government.

Contents

Figures

Tables

Summary

The past two decades have brought increasing awareness of the health effects of concussive brain injury, and a key driver of that awareness has been the blast-related injuries suffered during combat operations in Iraq and Afghanistan. There has been growing concern over the potential for subconcussive neurological injury after repeated low-level military occupational blast (MOB) exposures. Examples include heavy weapon and munition training (e.g., artillery, recoilless rifles, shoulder-mounted rocket launchers) and activities such as breaching.

The Seventh Department of Defense (DoD) State-of-the-Science Meeting (SoSM) was held March 12–15, 2018, at the RAND Corporation's offices in Arlington, Virginia. The meeting's theme was "The Neurological Effects of Repeated Exposure to Military Occupational Blast: Implications for Prevention and Health." These proceedings present (1) background on the SoSM, (2) results from a systematic literature review conducted in support of the SoSM, (3) the meeting's keynote address, (4) discussion panels and presentations, (5) working group findings, and (6) conclusions and recommendations compiled by the SoSM expert panel.

For the purpose of the SoSM, *MOB exposures* were defined as low-level blast exposures that do not result in loss of consciousness but for which repeated exposure may involve alteration of consciousness (also described as *subconcussive blast exposure*).

Researchers, clinicians, and military leaders from related fields attended the SoSM and provided overviews, presentations, and posters describing new and emerging science. Before the meeting, a multidisciplinary SoSM planning committee invited five leading scientists and clinicians to serve as an expert panel. Expert panelists led working groups and developed the overall SoSM recommendations. Working groups developed responses to four questions drafted in advance to address the meeting's objectives.

Immediately after the meeting, the SoSM expert panel, equipped with the findings of their respective working groups, convened to develop the research and policy recommendations for DoD. Summaries of the findings, discussed in more detail in Chapter Seven of these proceedings, were as follows:

The Secretary of Defense and senior military leaders should consider the following recommendations:

- **Recommendation 1.** Enforce DoD policies and standards related to low-level MOB exposure.
- **Recommendation 2.** Develop a research portfolio of high-quality studies assessing exposure to repeated, low-level occupational blast injury.
- **Recommendation 3.** Prepare and plan, in response to recent legislation, for a large-scale population-based longitudinal study of military personnel, with a long follow-up window to assess the prevalence and severity of neurological and general health outcomes after repeated, low-level MOB exposure.

- **Recommendation 4.** Continue an animal research portfolio of repeated, low-level blast exposure but emphasize experiments using larger animals, including nonhuman primate models, to facilitate the translation of findings to humans.
- **Recommendation 5.** Examine the potential neurologic and general health effects of low-level blast exposure indicators, comparing extant military exposure assessment tools and protective practices and devices when feasible and aligned with study objectives, to facilitate incremental improvements in safety and outcomes.
- **Recommendation 6.** Catalogue, map, and make available to researchers, safety programs, and military end users unclassified weapon system–specific information and service member–specific load profiles for key military occupations, exposures, and contexts.
- **Recommendation 7.** Design policies and increase opportunities for embedded scientists to study repeated MOB exposure in training units and deployed contexts.

Acknowledgments

We gratefully acknowledge Michael Leggieri, Raj Gupta, and COL Sidney Hinds of the Blast Injury Research Program Project Coordinating Office for their comments, guidance, and support for this project. We also recognize the extensive work that the office did prior to RAND's involvement, refining the SoSM process, which the office has used to develop DoD research policy and priorities related to blast injury since 2009.

We would also like to thank the stakeholders consulted on topic selection and the planning committee who provided invaluable guidance as we prepared for the meeting and the associated literature review. In addition, we are grateful to the meeting presenters, working group facilitators, and all of the attendees whose diverse views, thoughtful feedback, and commitment strengthened the meeting.

We thank Quiana Fulton, Benjamin N. Harris, Sara-Laure Faraji, William Mackenzie, and Nathan Vest for taking notes during the meeting; Mary Kate Adgie, Gina Frost, and Tandrea Parrot for their onsite administrative support; and Kevin Bynum, Leanna Shrader, and Mohammad Yasseen for their planning assistance. Finally, the meeting would not have been as successful without Kristin Sereyko's hard work and project management.

Abbreviations

BBB	blood-brain barrier
BrdU	bromodeoxyuridine
bTBI	blast-induced traumatic brain injury
CHRNA7	nicotinic/neuronal acetylcholine receptor, subunit $\alpha 7$
dB	decibel
DG	dentate gyrus
DoD	Department of Defense
DTI	diffusion tensor imaging
EMP	electromagnetic pulse
GFAP	glial fibrillary acidic protein
I-TAB	Investigating the Neurologic Effect of Training Associated Blast
kPa	kilopascal
MOB	military occupational blast
MRI	magnetic resonance imaging
mTBI	mild traumatic brain injury
PCS	postconcussive syndrome
PPE	personal protective equipment
psi	pounds per square inch
PTSD	posttraumatic stress disorder
RNA	ribonucleic acid
ROS	reactive oxygen species
SoSM	State-of-the-Science Meeting
SPB	sodium phenylbutyrate
TBI	traumatic brain injury
TCD	transcranial Doppler
TRPV1	transient receptor potential vanilloid 1
TUDCA	tauroursodeoxycholic acid
UCH-L1	ubiquitin carboxy-terminal hydrolase L1

VA   Department of Veterans Affairs

1. Background

The past two decades have brought heightened understanding and awareness of the health effects of concussive brain injury, also known as mild traumatic brain injury (mTBI). A key driver of that awareness has been the blast-related injuries suffered during combat operations in Iraq and Afghanistan. More recently, concern has grown over the potential for *sub*concussive neurological injury following repetitive exposure to common types of low-level military occupational blasts (MOBs). Examples may include heavy weapons training and use (e.g., artillery, recoilless rifles, shoulder-mounted rocket launchers) and activities such as breaching.

To address research policy priorities and gaps, the Seventh Department of Defense (DoD) State-of-the-Science Meeting (SoSM) was held March 12–15, 2018, at the RAND Corporation's offices in Arlington, Virginia. The meeting theme was "The Neurological Effects of Repeated Exposure to Military Occupational Levels of Blast: Implications for Health and Prevention."

These SoSM proceedings provide summary information on (1) the background on the SoSM; (2) a systematic literature review RAND Arroyo Center completed in support of the SoSM; (3) the SoSM keynote address; (4) SoSM discussion panels and presentations; (5) working group findings; and (6) SoSM conclusions and recommendations. For the purpose of the SoSM, *MOB exposures* were defined as low-level blast exposures that do not result in loss of consciousness but for which repeated exposure may involve alteration of consciousness (also described as *subconcussive blast exposure*).

To prepare for and inform the experts who participated in the SoSM, the DoD Blast Injury Research Program Coordinating Office asked RAND Arroyo Center to complete a systematic literature review on the potential neurological effects of repeated MOB exposure. The resulting literature review addressed specific questions that aligned with the SoSM objectives; the conclusions can be found in Chapter Two of these proceedings.

A 33-member, interagency planning committee was convened that included members from clinical and research communities representing the Army, Navy, Air Force, DoD, Department of Veterans Affairs (VA), academia, and nonprofits (see Appendix A). The role of the planning committee was to refine meeting objectives, provide consultation for the literature review, approve the SoSM agenda (see Appendix B), recommend the SoSM keynote speaker (see Appendix C) and discussion panel participants (see Appendix D), formulate working group questions (see Chapter Six), and review and prioritize submitted abstracts for scientific presentations versus posters (see Chapter Five and Appendix E). The planning committee also guided the selection of a five-member expert panel (see Appendix F). Expert panelists were charged with chairing working group sessions, and they developed and prioritized the major findings and recommendations.

More than 130 researchers, clinicians, policymakers, and military leaders from related disciplines attended the SoSM (see Appendix G) and were charged with participating in a working group. Under the leadership of an expert panelist, each working group developed consensus responses to questions designed to address the SoSM objectives:

- Describe blast exposures that are repeatedly incurred during military service.
- Describe the research into the potential neurological consequences and mechanisms of repeated blast exposure.
- Examine strategies for preventing injuries due to repeated MOBs.
- Identify indicators that may be used for early detection of health consequences of repeated blast exposure.
- Prioritize key research and policy gaps related to repeated MOB exposure and projects and initiatives to address them.

The consolidated outputs from the five working group sessions are presented in Chapter Six. Final SoSM recommendations are summarized in Chapter Seven. These recommendations are expected to guide future DoD-funded blast injury medical research policies and priorities.

2. Literature Review Summary

In preparation for the SoSM, the DoD Blast Injury Research Program Coordinating Office asked RAND Arroyo Center to conduct a review of recent research literature on neurological injury from low-level MOB exposure. **Charles Engel (RAND Corporation)** shared the literature review findings at the meeting.

MOB exposures were defined as low-level blast exposures that do not result in loss of consciousness but for which repeated exposure may involve alteration of consciousness. Repeated MOB exposure leads to subconcussive injuries but not mild or more severe traumatic brain injury (TBI).

The literature review addressed several specific research questions:

- What is known about the occurrence of repeated low-level blast exposure incurred during military service?
- What is the scientific evidence related to the potential neurological health effects?
- What are promising strategies for preventing neurological damage?
- What are promising indicators for early detection of potential neurological consequences?

Literature Review Methods

RAND researchers reviewed studies related to low-level MOB exposure to promote a shared understanding of the current evidence base on the short-, intermediate-, and long-term neurological outcomes. The review captured a range of important outcomes, including functional status, physical and emotional symptoms, neuropsychological outcomes, theoretically plausible biomarkers, and clinical injuries and illnesses. Human studies to date have largely focused on population samples exposed to blasts during combat, making it difficult to differentiate between primary blast injuries from repeated low-level MOB (i.e., those resulting from the blast overpressure wave) and secondary and tertiary blast injury effects (penetrating injuries from blast fragments and blunt force injuries when an individual is thrown by a blast, respectively). These studies were observational, with blast exposure assessed through self-reports, often months or years later. Animal studies offer the important advantages of experimental design for causal inference and the capacity to isolate the effects of blast overpressure, so the review included animal studies that evaluated primary blast exposures of 20 pounds per square inch (psi) or less. There are concerns in the scientific community about interspecies variation in blast effects—which challenge efforts to correlate blast levels in animals to those in humans—and interlaboratory measurement variation. However, to address questions of biological plausibility, in particular, we decided to include appropriate experimental animal evidence.

We used a three-step process to develop search terms. First, we identified potential search terms from previous DoD blast injury research state-of-the-science literature reviews, terms specifically relevant to the current topic, and related National Library of Medicine Medical

Subject Headings. Then, we performed a preliminary literature search and used the results to improve our search strategy. Finally, the planning committee, a group of experts from fields related to the study topic, reviewed the search terms and recommended additional terms and search modifications.

We then used a five-step process to produce this literature review: (1) we defined key questions; (2) we conducted a literature search; (3) we screened titles, abstracts, and full text of the search results; (4) we abstracted the data; and (5) we synthesized the remaining sources to develop the findings presented in this chapter. We also searched peer-reviewed and gray literature on the nature and effect of routinely incurring low levels of MOB exposure, including peer-reviewed scientific literature in PubMed, Web of Science, and PsycINFO, as well as research reports and proposals in the Defense Technical Information Center database, dating from 2007 to 2017. We identified additional relevant publications from bibliographies of articles, targeted searches, and planning committee recommendations. Eligible studies included related human and animal studies and bioengineering models. These proceedings present a review of findings from the 254 articles that met the final inclusion and exclusion criteria.

Literature Review Findings

Occurrence of Low-Level MOB Exposure

We identified no research on the overall frequency with which low-level MOB occurs. There have been a handful of studies evaluating potentially informative populations such as explosive breachers, shoulder-mounted artillery operators, and military service members deployed and in training. There are few if any guidelines or models that could be used to determine a safe level of MOB exposure at the low per-occurrence levels common in training or analogous settings.

Potential Neurologic Effects of Low-Level MOB

We identified no human or animal studies revealing specific motor effects of low-level MOB exposure and no human studies revealing neurosensory effects of low-level MOB exposure. A study of rats exposed to low-level blasts found increased expression of the pain mediator transient receptor potential vanilloid 1 (TRPV1) in corneal tissue. Although we identified no human studies revealing persistent cognitive effects of low-level MOB, a number of studies in rats and mice suggest that the cognitive domain may be particularly sensitive to low-level blast. In these animal studies, blast exposures ranging from 3 to 10 psi were associated with reduced learning or cognition persisting up to 30 days.

We identified no human studies of neuropathology related to low-level MOB, based on our definition. Published studies have exclusively focused on combat samples with higher-level blast exposure. A number of studies have used rats and mice, however. Findings from these studies include evidence of increased permeability of the blood-brain barrier (BBB) on magnetic resonance imaging (MRI); increases in fractional anisotropy; decreases in radial diffusivity on diffusion tensor imaging (DTI); changes to the cortex and hippocampus; white-matter changes, including greater amyloid precursor protein immunoreactive cells; chronic microvascular changes; scattered pyknotic neurons; altered gene expression after low-level blast; dynamic microglial and macrophage responses; and microdomains of brain microvascular dysfunction.

Behavioral and Emotional

Cross-sectional human studies have suggested that symptoms of blast-related TBI may be largely explained by coexisting posttraumatic stress disorder (PTSD) and depression. However, other cross-sectional studies suggest that blast exposure may increase PTSD arousal symptoms (e.g., hypervigilance). Some researchers have hypothesized, based on animal studies, that blast exposure may unmask arousal symptoms by reducing frontal lobe inhibition of the amygdala, a center of fear expression previously implicated in PTSD and thought to heighten psychological threat response.

Auditory and Vestibular

We identified research showing an association between low-level MOB exposure and auditory/vestibular impairments and symptoms in combat-deployed service members as well as in an animal study. Exposure to low-level blast from small-caliber firearms is associated with middle-ear dysfunction—even when wearing earplugs—and may play a role in the early stage of auditory fatigue leading to tinnitus. The vestibular system helps maintain balance and postural stability and could be affected by repeated exposure to low-level blasts, though these effects are not well understood.

Visual

We identified no human studies detailing effects on the eye from low-level MOB exposure. Closed-globe eye injuries are known to result from combat-related blast exposure, although these injuries typically occur at higher blast levels than those that were the focus of this review. Evidence in rats suggests that single and repeated low-level blast exposure may lead to increased pain and inflammation in corneal tissue.

Early Exposure Indicators

Studies in animals and humans have examined a variety of biomarkers, with inconsistent findings to date. Preliminary studies of biosensors to monitor troops for concussive effects after blast exposure have so far proved disappointing, and we found no studies that used biosensor data to assess subconcussive blast.

Potential Prevention

The review captured several preventive methods, including barrier and nonbarrier methods and safety guidelines. Research on barrier methods has included helmets, earplugs, and body armor. Helmets (e.g., the Advanced Combat Helmet) are typically designed to protect the wearer from head trauma due to projectiles rather than blast exposure and may sometimes even amplify blast exposure. Earplugs are the most effective barrier protection from hearing-related blast injury. The limited research on nonbarrier prevention methods suggests that education programs may increase the use of hearing protection.

Literature Review Responses to Questions

What Is Known About the Occurrence of Repeated Low-Level Blast Exposure Incurred During Military Service?

The literature review found no published information on military service–specific frequencies of exposure to low-level MOB. The only information pertains to higher levels of blast exposure encountered in combat settings.

What Is the Scientific Evidence Related to the Potential Neurological Health Effects?

Experimental studies in animals suggest that persistent neurological effects from low-level blast exposure (i.e., under 10 psi) are plausible. However, interspecies differences in exposure susceptibility may be large, and there have been no experimental studies of low-level blast effects in nonhuman primates. Hence, there remains significant uncertainty as to how low-level blast exposure effects observed in animal studies translate to humans.

Epidemiologic and clinical studies of military personnel provide sufficient evidence of an association among combat-related blast exposure without penetrating injury, postconcussive syndrome (PCS), and PTSD. However, these blast exposure levels are higher than the subconcussive exposures of interest in this review, blast exposures of a level occurring during routine field training, breaching, artillery fire, and shoulder-mounted weapon discharge. Moreover, the precise nature of the relationship between PCS and PTSD remains unclear. It is possible that nonspecific symptoms of PTSD may explain the apparent association between low-level blast and PCS.

What Are Promising Strategies for Preventing Neurological Damage?

Prevention programs targeting health risks that do not exist or implementing methods that are not effective are clearly a waste of societal resources that can be put to more productive use in other ways. Therefore, the relevance of discussions regarding prevention strategies depends on the answers to several key questions that remain unanswered:

- *Is low-level MOB a significant risk to current and future force health?* To devote significant resources to preventing the negative health effects of an exposure, there should be consensus—ideally, based on empirical data—that the threat to health is significant.
- *Are current preventive interventions safe and effective?* Even if the problem is substantial, ineffective primary prevention approaches will prove wasteful.

- *Will preventive intervention benefits outweigh the harms*? If a preventive intervention is effective but renders the population vulnerable to more serious threats, then implementation would be self-defeating.
- *Is the preventive intervention timely and feasible?* If the preventive intervention is perfectly effective but cannot be delivered in time, it is not useful. There are any number of related factors to consider here, such as the availability of relevant materials and staffing, as well as the acceptability of the intervention among leaders, service members, and the larger society.

Given the early state of the research into low-level MOB as a problem distinct from blast-related TBI, we recommend a cautious approach that would complete the research into the effects of preventive intervention development and testing before implementing aggressive, organization-wide surveillance and prevention programs specifically targeting low-level MOB.

Current protective measures against high-intensity combat blast injuries (e.g., mild, moderate, and severe TBI) should continue to be used. However, as it pertains to the effect of these and other protective measures for low-level MOB, the state of the science is preliminary at best.

What Are Promising Indicators for Early Detection of Potential Neurological Consequences?

We were unable to identify early detection biomarkers, a key type of early detection indicator, in humans. Even candidate biomarkers remain highly speculative and less than feasible, as they are exclusively the product of rat and mouse studies. Biosensors are a second key indicator, but we were similarly unable to identify published biosensor studies designed to assess the health effects of low-level MOB. The development and validation of improved human biosensor systems and methods of using human biosensor data to model the physiologic and physical effects of low-level MOB on human tissue should be prioritized and pursued. Biosensor data is potentially a low-burden method for modeling low-level MOB exposure for use in prospective cohort research designs.

Literature Review Summary

The most striking finding from this review of the literature was the lack of research and understanding of the organizational threat and service member health impact of low-level MOB—an understanding necessarily distinct from and in contrast to our rapidly improving understanding of blast-related mTBI. The National Defense Authorization Act for Fiscal Year 2018 included a requirement to design, initiate, and complete a prospective longitudinal cohort study of low-level MOB in a population-based sample of service members that would help fill this gap. The recommendations in this chapter center on the need to improve understanding of low-level MOB through a coordinated program of epidemiologic, etiologic, measurement, and preventive intervention research rather than resource-intensive or organization-wide efforts to implement population exposure surveillance.

3. Keynote Address

MG Malcolm Frost, commanding general of the Center for Initial Military Training, Army Training and Doctrine Command, delivered the keynote address. Frost is a seasoned infantry officer who is responsible for preparing 120,000 new recruits for service annually. He opened the address with an overview of Army Training and Doctrine Command's role in training and leading the Army's Holistic Health and Fitness program, as tasked in the Army Campaign Plan. It blends physical and emotional health and incorporates medical, fitness, and lifestyle professionals down to the tactical level. The system addresses the increase in nondeployable numbers and medical issues facing soldiers.

Frost urged new research to address gaps in training to understand the effects of concussive events. There is neither baseline exposure history nor the ability to document repeated exposures. Despite tests of mental aptitude and ability to meet physical standards, there are no focused neurological assessments to establish a baseline for cognitive function. Additionally, the military does not measure variations in risk based on military occupational skill, risks resulting from exposure to pressure or sounds, or the potential impact of blast exposure. There is also a lack of awareness of safe minimum distances, safe maximum exposure levels, or when a safety threshold has been crossed.

Frost recommended original research that definitively shows whether cumulative low-level blast exposures cause degenerative brain disease or other health issues. He expressed concern that service members may be suffering from behavioral health problems and may not realize it. The lack of a tool for commanders to assess risk limits their ability to make informed decisions. Beyond wearing ear protection to prevent hearing loss, artillery commanders do not think about exposure to the "boom" or the effect of cumulative exposure. Frost emphasized that any formal references, guidance, or tools developed must be easily understood and used by field commanders.

4. Discussion Panels

Panel on Strategy: DoD Policy and Requirements

Each panelist presented a different approach to low-level blast exposure—focused on operations, research, policy, engineering, or public health—but all agreed that further research was needed to understand negative health outcomes and protect service members from unnecessary exposure. Building actionable solutions first requires better definitions of the problem. **LTC James McKnight (Army Medical Research and Materiel Command, Military Operational Medicine Research Program)** moderated the panel and opened the discussion by asking, "How do we balance the need for realistic combat training while simultaneously reducing potential training risks? Should the military consider alternative methods to train service members, such as virtual reality?" Impediments to data collection were a recurring theme throughout the discussion and limit research in several ways. First, there is the difficulty of measuring the strength of a blast. Weapon systems are tested in the middle of a field, where the only reflective system is the ground. However, in reality, blasts are usually fired behind a barrier, such as a wall, that will affect blast overpressure and impulse noise. Second, virtual reality is a limited replacement for training. When research results are collected, they should be shared early and widely with political and field leadership, something that is not always occurring.

The panel discussed several aspects of blast injury and the exposure data necessary for timely and appropriate changes to current practice. **James Zheng (Army Program Executive Office–Soldier)** explained that a challenge in developing personal protective equipment (PPE) is determining whether injury information is correlated with the threat. Without accurate readings, manufacturers and military leaders cannot respond to requirements. Some blast limits have been codified, such as the allowable number of rounds per 24-hour period. Nevertheless, some military members in attendance suggested that these requirements are not well incorporated into material fielding plans or shared with field commanders. Furthermore, such limits may not reflect the operating environment.

The panel and audience advised several ways forward. First, science must be part of the solution. To break the silos described here, researchers should be embedded within units. Second, metrics must be standardized. Currently, blast exposure limits are often conveyed by word of mouth, and there is poor alignment between training and combat environments. Third, opportunities to incorporate brain safety measures into occupational guidance should be pursued. Fourth, it is important to liaise with such groups as the Joint Prevention Medicine Policy Working Group and each of the services. Finally, *TBI* is an overused blanket term for head injuries. A more specific term for subconcussive injuries should be adopted.

Before any sentinel surveillance system is proposed, better data are needed to correlate the injury to the threat. For example, to what extent do overpressure, pulse, and noise lead to injury, and what type of PPE will protect exposed service members? Beyond cognitive tests, head injury tests need to be quantified and standardized as a first step toward biological surveillance of chronic outcome measures. Additionally, planners should recall that *allowable number of rounds* is a training concept and does not capture the number of small blasts a service member is exposed to in battle.

Panel on the State of Current Research and Solutions

There is an inherent risk when a service member puts on the uniform. It is important to accept that some blast exposure necessarily occurs. The challenge is in determining what dose is safe for successful military training, as well as what doses are harmful. These findings can then inform decisions about what level and frequency should be considered a blast event for which a service member may be rested or triaged to medical care. This panel promoted a fresh perspective on two broad themes: blast characterization and early warning indicators. The call for a medical longitudinal study in the National Defense Authorization Act for Fiscal Year 2018 is unnecessarily restricted to cognitive factors. Ocular, auditory, biological, and physiological studies can be added as well. The combination of these indicators will build a robust early warning system.

Grace Hwang (Johns Hopkins University Applied Physics Laboratory) moderated the panel and opened the discussion by commenting that the field is in its infancy when it comes to understanding the neurological effects of low-level occupational blast in humans. There is a vast amount of research on TBI, but all of it focuses on much higher blast levels. Similar to the policy panel, each speaker approached the state of the current science from a different discipline. There was general agreement that limited epidemiological data are available from which to draw inferences. Small case-controlled studies of breachers and military law enforcement personnel are available. Breachers are service members and civilian law enforcement professionals who use mechanical, ballistic, explosive, or thermal tools to enter or clear locked or barricaded structures. The Army is now employing larger studies to observe barely noticeable differences in neurological outcomes that are inconsistent across individuals. **Ibolja Cernak (STARR-C [Stress, Trauma and Resilience Research Consulting] LLC)** described her research on Kosovar soldiers, many of whom experienced such profound short-term memory deficits during combat operations in the 1990s that they could no longer function effectively. Cernak argued that such injuries start as functional, psychological, and cognitive impairments before showing on MRIs, emphasizing why investigations should not be exclusive to head trauma. **Vassillis Koliatsos (Johns Hopkins University School of Medicine)** described how axons are mechanically and hypoxically metabolically vulnerable. There is often a geographic coexistence of axonal injury and brain lesions. Consistent with Cernak's remarks, Koliatsos maintained that studies must move beyond regarding the brain as an isolated organ and incorporate examination of psychological, adjustment, pain, and other disorders.

Hwang asked, "What is the best way to define low-level blast? What levels of blast do weapon systems produce that service members train on?" There are three tiers of overpressure field measurements with wearable instrumentation. The vast majority measured below 2 psi or between 2 and 4 psi, both below the safety threshold on most ranges. Around 8 psi, there is a transition from low-level blast exposure to a level associated with diagnosable injury. However, these are single-dose measurements. Current sensors are not equipped to measure cumulative effects, such as a service member who experiences numerous 2-psi blasts in a routine training day. A new combined metric may be needed to capture frequency, impulse, and overpressure. Peak pressure is a useful proxy measure for a dose but lacks the sensitivity to track cumulative effects.

There was a discussion of the congressionally mandated longitudinal study of low-level MOB, addressing two related questions: (1) How should this study be designed, and which disciplines should be included, and (2) what models for similar studies exist? For example, are there lessons learned from the DoD Millennium Cohort or the Air Force Health (Ranch Hand) studies? There was consensus that replication of human studies is difficult. Experimental models are valuable only if they represent real-world problems. Panelists urged a cohort study over mass surveillance. A cohort study would allow researchers to follow service members after they leave active or reserve military duty, link medical records, incorporate professional and lifestyle exposure (e.g., sports injuries), and leverage opportunistic technology. Ideally, such a study would start with biomarker collection and neuroimaging at the start of service, but this would be difficult and costly to implement for all service members using a program of mass surveillance.

5. Scientific Presentation Summaries

After the keynote speech and discussion panel sessions, government and academic speakers delivered scientific presentations describing the state of the science and addressing related policy questions.

Understanding Potential Neurological Consequences and Mechanisms of Repeated Blast Exposure

CDR Josh Duckworth (Uniformed Services University) spoke about the gap in understanding of clinical and physiological responses to subconcussive blast exposure. The Combat and Training Queryable Exposure/Event Repository (CONQUER) is an epidemiological study of impact and acceleration events among service members. Duckworth provided an overview of six years of research looking at load and blast exposure in training scenarios. In three years, an instructor at a weapon school will cumulatively experience between 400 and 600 psi from shoulder-mounted artillery and other sources. Figure 5.1 shows how even those who do not fire a heavy weapon may still incur some amount of overpressure. The Neurocognitive Assessment of Blast Exposure Sequelae in Training study found significant deficits in memory, learning, and executive function in 20 percent of a sample of Navy SEALs and Marines who participated in shoulder-fired weapon training.

Figure 5.1. Typical Blast Overpressure Map for Shoulder-Fired Heavy Weapons

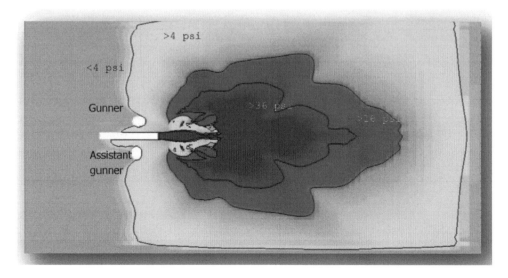

SOURCE: Duckworth, 2018.

Ongoing research includes the Investigating the Neurologic Effect of Training Associated Blast (I-TAB) study, which is measuring clinical and physiologic variability associated with repeated sub-concussive blast exposure. Preliminary findings recorded temporal changes in micro ribonucleic acid (RNA) expression associated with blast exposure. Five biomarkers were studied in serum after exposure: GFAP (glial fibrillary acidic protein), UCH-L1 (ubiquitin carboxy-terminal hydrolase L1), CHRNA7 (nicotinic/neuronal acetylcholine receptor, subunit α7), Claudin-5, and occuldin. Differences in serums between students and instructors are shown in Figure 5.2. Duckworth indicated that future research should seek to quantify relationships between blast exposure and physiologic processes and to provide insights that can guide leader recommendations to remove individual service members or return them to duty.

Figure 5.2. I-TAB Preliminary Findings in Brain Serum

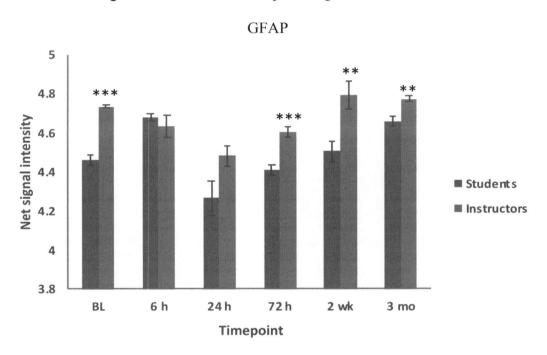

UCH-L1

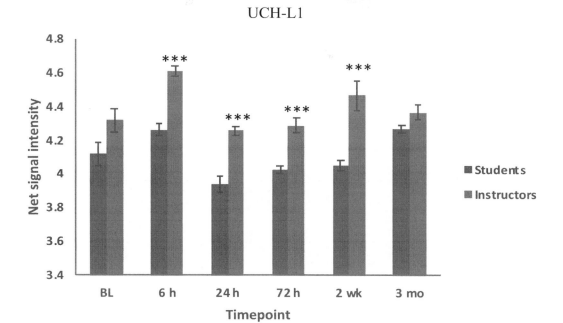

CHRNA7

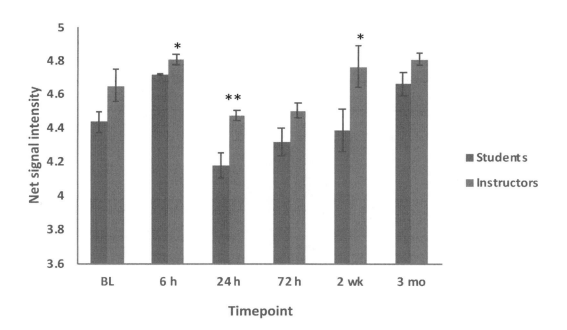

Claudin-5

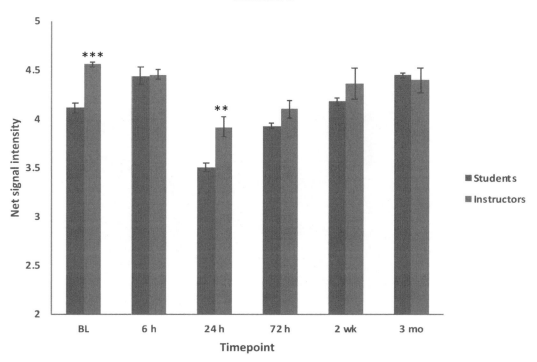

Occludin

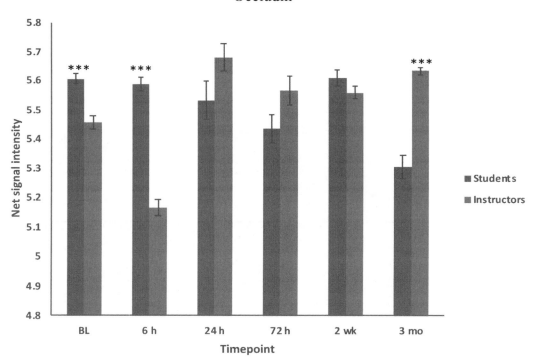

SOURCE: Duckworth, 2018.
NOTE: Instructor (10) vs. student (6); student's t-test; * $p < 0.05$; ** $p < 0.01$; *** $p < 0.0001$.

Profiling of Blast-Overpressure Effects on the Human Brain in Breacher Training

Jia Lu (DSO National Laboratories) addressed profiling of blast-overpressure effects on the human brain in breacher training. There is no scientific basis for how close is too close to a blast or what cumulative level, frequency, or time frame for exposure is dangerous. The true operational burden and long-term risks of what those who experience it call "breacher brain" are unknown. Breacher brain essentially represents a collection of symptoms reported by people regularly exposed to subconcussive blasts, such as fatigue, memory loss, headaches, and slowed thought processes (Shanker and Oppel, 2014).

To move from anecdotal reporting of symptoms and to start answering questions about how blast exposure relates to various outcomes, an analogue to the Bowen curve designed for neurologic injury is needed. Classic Bowen curves are empirically derived and based on many experiments in which animals are exposed to a blast wave. After blast exposure is delivered under various conditions, it is noted whether the animal survives or dies within 24 hours. By exposing many animals to the same blast load, a ratio of how many animals die within 24 hours as a function of peak blast overpressure and the duration of the positive overpressure wave can be assessed (Teland, 2012). To date, Bowen-style curves have not been developed to model the occurrence of brain injury under different environmental conditions (e.g., an enclosure, near a concrete wall, in an open field) and varying blast wave conditions (a range of peak overpressures and positive overpressure wave duration). The challenges to developing these models for repetitive low-level occupational blast are great, particularly for subjective symptom-based outcomes.

Lu went on to present data from Singapore Armed Forces breachers in which personnel wore blast gauges and completed the Automated Neuropsychological Assessment Metric to examine short-term cognitive changes. Healthy male soldiers were profiled during 15 live-fire exercises over three years. In 32 blast events, blast overpressure rarely exceeded 2 psi. Figure 5.3 indicates the areas of the brain where one might plausibly expect changes that would affect behavior or memory (e.g., anterior cingulate, cerebellum, hippocampus). However, using the Automated Neuropsychological Assessment Metric, Lu's team did not observe any functional or cognitive changes in the one-month study, nor did MRI or biomarker tests express any gross or macroscopic changes.

Figure 5.3. Brain Regions Vulnerable to Blast Injury (circled in red)

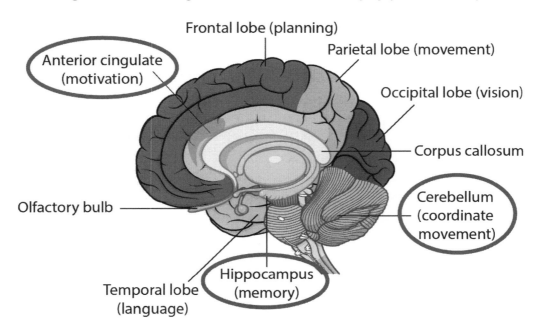

Quantifying Occupational Blast Exposure During Military and Law Enforcement Training

Gary Kamimori (Walter Reed Army Institute of Research) spoke on quantifying occupational blast exposure during military and law enforcement training. He described several field experiments, reminding the audience, "Blast in the lab is *not* the same as operational blast. Scientists need to be exposed to what operators are exposed to." Kamimori emphasized the importance of accurately measuring incident versus reflective overpressure and sensor orientation, as well as completely capturing the blast wave. Agreed-upon definitions of blast and pressure are necessary to evaluate risk. Kamimori proposed the following:

- When the reflecting surface is parallel to the blast wave, the minimum *incident pressure* will be experienced.
- When the shock wave impinges on a surface that is perpendicular to the direction it is traveling, the point of impact will experience the maximum *reflected pressure*.

For example, if one were to punch someone in the face, everything leading up to the initial contact is incident pressure and everything after contact is reflective pressure. Table 5.1 provides a reference for the different intensity of blasts that a service member can experience and the effects on humans and structures.

Table 5.1. PSI: Injury and Structural Damage Thresholds

Pressure		Effect on Human (1-microsecond pulse duration)	Effect on Structure
psi	kPa		
0.3	2	140 dB (noise limit for unprotected hearing)	
0.5	3		Windows break
1	7		Studs and drywall crack
2	14		
3	20		Structural damage begins
4	28		Reinforced concrete walls crack
5	34	Threshold for eardrum rupture (15%)	
6	41		Collapse of wood frame structure
7	48		
8	54		Reinforced concrete wall displaced
9	61		
10	68		Shattered automotive glass, damaged buildings collapse
15	102	50% chance of eardrum rupture	
20	136		Reinforced concrete walls destroyed
30	204	Threshold for lung injury	
40	272		
50	340		4.5 ft from 50-lb bare explosive
100	680	Slight chance of death (pulmonary-related)	
150	1,020	50% chance of death (pulmonary-related)	
200	1,360	100% chance of death (pulmonary-related)	2.5 ft from 50-lb bare explosive

SOURCE: Kamimori, 2018.

Kamimori described several experiments characterizing overpressure exposure, demonstrating how the level of blast experienced varies by the type and angle of the charge and crew position. For example, in one experiment with a M119 105-mm howitzer, the chief of section experienced nearly 50 percent more peak overpressure, 2.0 psi, than the loader, who experienced 1.3 psi. A separate experiment at Fort Benning, Georgia, involved 81-mm (M252) and 120-mm (M120) mortars and four-member crews, plus a range safety officer. It measured peak and impulse overpressure using four blast sensors mounted to each helmet. Similar to the howitzer experiment, each team member was exposed to a different amount of blast and impulse overpressure, and instructors reported symptoms consistent with PCS without actually experiencing a concussion (i.e., breacher brain). Because operators are rarely in an open field and exposed to a single blast wave, future experiments must look at close-quarters training and potential links between blast pressure and acoustics.

Receiving a Multiple Peak Blast Dose in a Single Complex Blast Event

Jean-Philippe Dionne (Med-Eng) shared the results of several experiments involving municipal police department breaching teams. He showed how a series of successive blasts could have a cumulative effect, eventually surpassing a biological threshold and resulting in significant adverse central nervous system effects.

The Friedlander waveform shown in Figure 5.4 is used to model blast overpressure once a blast is fully developed and assumes no nearby reflective surfaces. In the real world, reflective surfaces are present, complex, and may amplify blast effects. As a result, the ideal Friedlander waveform serves only as an approximation of the actual "messy" blast exposure (Figure 5.5). In addition, the pathological effects of the blast on the central nervous system are cumulative; with each successive blast, the peak pressure necessary to affect the nervous system lessens. Dionne's work is developing calculations and curves that can be used to estimate the real-world effects of blast waves on the brain. Despite the use of isolated blasts in ideal conditions, these experiments allow the development of engineering models and materials for measuring complex blasts in real-world conditions.

Figure 5.4. Schematic of an Ideal Friedlander Waveform

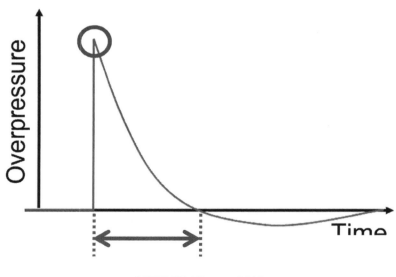

SOURCE: Dionne, 2018.

NOTE: Peak overpressure occurs in the blue circle, and the duration of the positive overpressure wave is the interval of time, delineated in green. The positive overpressure wave is followed by an interval of negative overpressure, during which the observed pressure is less than the original baseline pressure (shown below the x-axis).

Figure 5.5. Example of a Single Messy Blast Dose

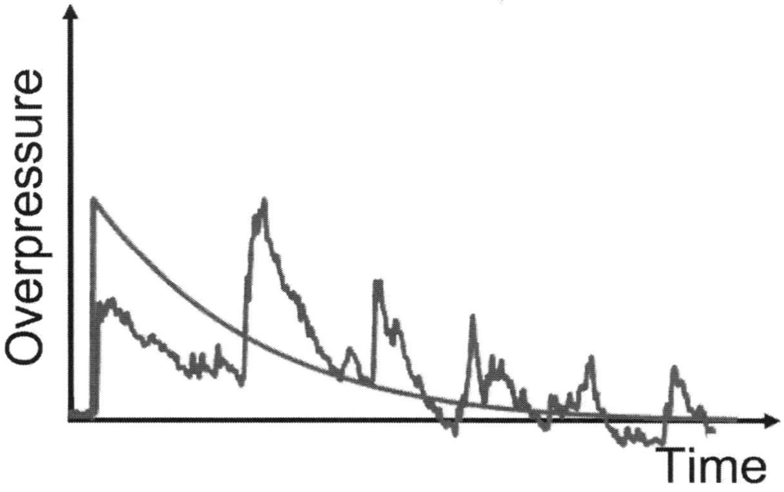

SOURCE: Dionne, 2018.

Suicide in Combatants with Extensive Blast Exposure: Strictly a Mental Health Issue or Evidence of Underlying Structural Brain Lesions?

Daniel Perl (Uniformed Services University) presented three recent cases of suicide in former Navy SEALs. Pathologic investigation of each service member's brain revealed patterns of interface glial scarring. All three service members had several blast exposures in training and in combat, though they were not injured severely enough for a medical referral. All three had also suffered from PTSD and prominent neurologic behavior syndrome, including headaches, sleep disturbances, anxiety, memory problems, and mood swings. Perl hypothesized that repeated blast exposure accompanied by brain lesions can induce behaviors conducive to patients committing suicide. He urged researchers to examine suicide not only as a mental health issue but also as the result of an interaction between structural abnormalities and psychological health factors.

Impaired Stress Coping and Cognitive Function Caused by Blast Exposure

Ibolja Cernak (STARR-C [Stress, Trauma and Resilience Research and Consulting] LLC) illustrated the typical timeline of blast injuries and resulting impaired stress coping and cognitive function. For blast loading injuries, the time to peak force and pressure occurs over less than 100 microseconds. For comparison, the average human eye blink takes 350,000 microseconds. Blunt impact and ballistic injuries typically take much longer. Even though sports concussions can also lead to neurodegeneration, the physics of impact is markedly different. Figure 5.6 shows the typical timeline for blast, ballistic, and blunt injuries.

Figure 5.6. Typical Timeline of Blast, Ballistic, and Blunt Injuries Compared with Ergonomics-Related Injuries Based on the Duration of Peak Force

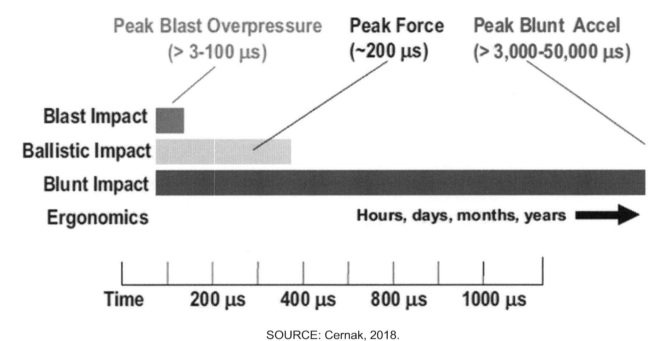

SOURCE: Cernak, 2018.

In a typical explosion, a high-explosive shock wave strikes a living body and a number of events take place. First, the body does not absorb the entire shock wave. A fraction is reflected, and a fraction propagates through the body as tissue-transmitted pressure waves. Second, two types of tissue response are observed. One is caused by the impulse of the shock wave and one by the pressure variations in the form of oscillations or pressure deflections. Injury from repeated exposure to low-level blast starts early with functional deficits, and, if tracked over time, clinicians and researchers may observe neurodegeneration. Figure 5.7 maps the consequences of tissue-transmitted pressure propagation.

Figure 5.7. Consequences of Tissue-Transmitted Pressure Propagation

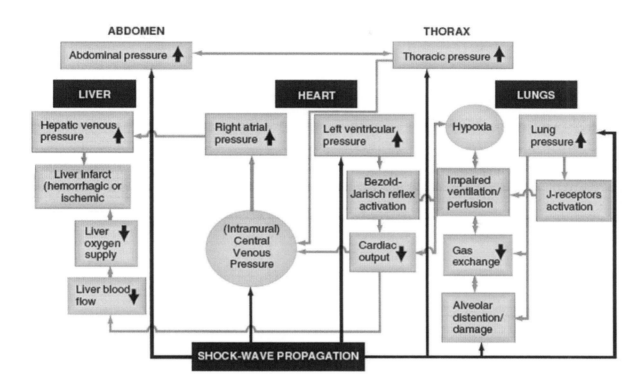

SOURCE: Institute of Medicine, 2014, p. 42, Figure 3-4.

Cernak argued that if researchers know what symptoms are attributable to low-level occupational blast, they can start early by tracking functional deficits and progression based on markers for neurodegeneration. A study of Canadian service members (n = 116) found a broad range of neuroendocrine and immune system changes, as well as impaired cognitive function, in those exposed to blast. A description of these changes is presented in Table 5.2.

Table 5.2. Blast-Induced Neurotrauma

Acute/Sub-Acute Neurotrauma (impaired neurologic functions; potentially reversible)	Chronic Neurotrauma (impaired brain tissue integrity; irreversible)
Cognitive deficits	Necrotic and apoptotic cell death in the brain
Increased BBB permeability	Long-term neurological deficits
Diffusion and perfusion deficits	Irreversible diffuse axonal damage
Diffuse axonal damages	Neurogenic inflammation
Failure of energy metabolism	

SOURCE: Cernak, 2018.

Occupational Risk Moderates the Relationship Between Major Blast Exposure and Traumatic Brain Injury

Jennifer N. Belding (Naval Health Research Center) studied whether the likelihood of developing a TBI after a major blast depended on the amount of chronic overpressure to which service members are exposed. Using the Post-Deployment Health Assessment, a sample of more than 180,000 active-duty Marines, researchers categorized respondents into Marine occupational specialties and then organized those personnel into occupations they expected were at more versus less risk of blast exposure (see Table 5.3). They found that the likelihood of screening positive for TBI on the Post-Deployment Health Assessment was separately related to (1) self-reported blast exposure and (2) prior high-risk occupation. Furthermore, screening positive for TBI was most common among those with both of these factors.

Belding asserted that one explanation for the finding is the presence of a priming effect (repeated low-level occupational exposures among those in high-blast-risk occupations may have increased their vulnerability to subsequent concussive blast injuries). The researchers plan to explore self-reported symptomology and persistence of symptoms to look for evidence suggesting a similar potential priming effect on recovery (i.e., that those in high-blast-risk occupations and with concussive blast exposure who develop postconcussive symptoms may take the longest to recover). Future studies will have to investigate a range of confounders, such as proximity to the blast, number of blasts, and recreational exposures, for example, from sports injuries. To improve epidemiological investigations, Belding urged that records capture specific job descriptions, field exercises, and behavioral health so they can be linked to data from VA records to assess longitudinal outcomes.

Table 5.3. High- and Low-Risk Marine Occupational Specialties

Low-Blast-Risk Occupations	High-Blast-Risk Occupations
Communications	Ammunition and explosive ordnance disposal
Financial management	Aircraft maintenance
Food service	Airfield services
Legal services	Combat camera
Meteorology and oceanography	Field artillery
Music	Infantry
Personnel and administration	Tank and amphibious assault vehicle
Public affairs	

SOURCE: Belding, 2018.

Epidemiologic Study of Occupational Blast Exposure and Subsequent Diagnoses

MAJ Walter Carr (Center for Military Psychiatry and Neuroscience, Walter Reed Army Institute of Research) presented an epidemiology of occupational blast exposure. He hypothesized a cause and effect between blast exposure and neurological outcomes. In a 2008 field study of Marines at Quantico, a survey of self-reported symptoms lacked questions specific enough to determine a causal link. A new pilot study will address some of these gaps by asking more specific questions about blast intensity and type of ordnance. In addition, the earlier study found that all of the outcome variables were subclinical, so medical records were less useful. Service members are not pulled off the firing line for exposure to these blasts. A later substudy of existing records and a matched cohort cross-sectional study found that, by virtue of their occupation, artillery soldiers may be exposed to hundreds of rounds per year, with each round achieving 1–2 psi peak pressure. The only significant difference between cohorts was the prevalence of tinnitus; however, instructors reported losing their balance or posture after blast exposure. Future studies will need to target the central nervous system and enhance the ability to measure physical changes in soldiers. In addition, soldiers practicing on the firing range may choose not to access medical care, limiting the reliability of a study based on medical records.

Blast-Induced "PTSD": Evidence from an Animal Model

Greg Elder (James J. Peters VA Medical Center/Icahn School of Medicine at Mount Sinai) presented evidence from an animal model of blast-induced "PTSD." Blast exposure without other psychological trauma can induce a PTSD-like state. Whereas TBI is a physical injury, PTSD is a syndrome induced by a psychological stressor. Moderate to severe TBI is recognizable by cognitive defects, but mTBI and PTSD have overlapping symptoms.

A study using rat models found that a blast could induce PTSD-related behavioral traits, such as anxiety response or acoustic startle, in the absence of a psychological stressor. Rats were tested six and eight months after three exposures to 75-kPa (~10.8 psi) blasts. In both instances, rats exhibited an anxiety response. Prior blast exposure may induce a priming effect, making animals more likely to react abnormally to a subsequent psychological stressor. Pathological review of brains in both groups found an accumulation of glial tau in the anterior cortex and hippocampus, which mimicked features of human tauopathy. Several of the overlapping symptoms are in Figure 5.8.

Figure 5.8. Overlapping Symptoms of PCS and PTSD

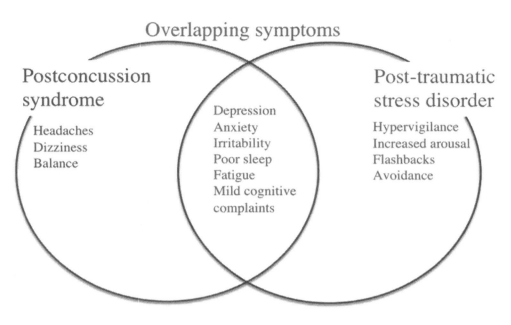

Overlapping symptoms

Postconcussion syndrome

Headaches
Dizziness
Balance

Depression
Anxiety
Irritability
Poor sleep
Fatigue
Mild cognitive
complaints

Post-traumatic stress disorder

Hypervigilance
Increased arousal
Flashbacks
Avoidance

SOURCE: Elder, 2018.

The Dynamics of Structural Changes After Repeated Mild Blast TBI: Acute Pathologies and Lasting Consequences

Denes Agoston (Uniformed Services University) spoke on the structural and molecular changes to the brain after repeated exposure to mild blast. Trainees are routinely exposed to blasts during training exercises. Seventy percent of affected soldiers are between 20 and 34 years old, a neurodevelopmentally vulnerable age. Agoston tested the cumulative effect of repeated exposure using rat models in a blast tube. With the rats in the blast tube unrestrained with lateral exposure, each subject was exposed to three 15.5- to 19.4-psi blasts 30 minutes apart. In an effort to compare rats to humans, rat brains were examined three months post-exposure, a period representing 15 percent of their lifespan. Using a combination of DTI analysis and measured parameters—volume, fractional anisotropy, axial diffusivity, radial diffusivity, and apparent diffusion coefficient—allowed a more comprehensive view of the injury process than earlier studies. Three major findings were as follows: (1) an evolving repeated mild blast-induced TBI pathology, (2) brain regions showing differential vulnerability, and (3) an altered trajectory of late-stage neurodevelopment. Repeated mild blast exposure caused long-term changes in the volume of specific gray- and white-matter functions. Structural imbalances in the brain have functional consequences for such areas as memory and executive function, key functions in an operating environment.

Neuronal Response to Multiple Shock Tube Overpressure Exposures

Thomas O'Shaughnessy (Naval Research Laboratory) looked at neuronal responses to multiple shock tube overpressure exposures. Inserting four neuronal cultures into an anthropomorphic head system (see Figure 5.9), the team looked for a dose response relationship between peak overpressure and cell metabolism.

Figure 5.9. Anthropomorphic Head System

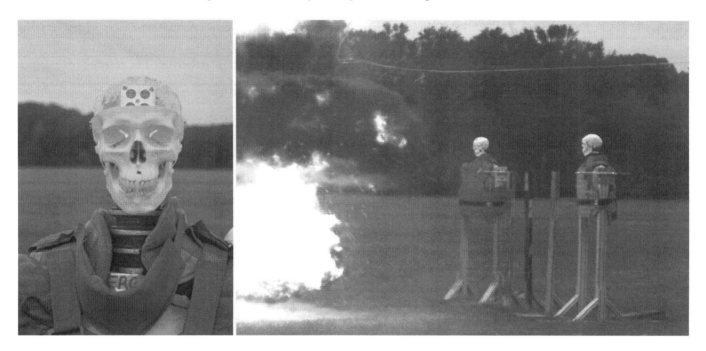

SOURCE: O'Shaughnessy, 2018.

Over four days, there was a statistically significant progressive decrease in metabolism versus controls. This research concluded that repeated overpressure exposure can produce further decreases in cell culture metabolism relative to the first exposure. Based on these results, O'Shaughnessy and team hypothesized that the initial overpressure insult may activate a metabolic cellular pathway that renders the cells more susceptible to a second and subsequent impacts.

Blood-Brain Barrier Permeability Is a Sensitive Neurological Marker for Single and Repeated Occupational Low-Level Blast Exposures in a Rodent Model

Namas Chandra (New Jersey Institute of Technology) presented work to develop a preclinical rodent model for assessing the relationship of blast characteristics (e.g., peak overpressure, duration of the positive phase of overpressure) to evidence of increased permeability of the BBB. He hypothesizes that BBB permeability is a sensitive neurological marker for single and repeated low-level occupational blast exposure. Much of Chandra's work relies on placing rodents into a "shock tube," exposing the animals to controlled sequences of one or more blasts, and assessing behavioral and physiologic outcomes. He indicated that there is significant variation in the shock tube models carried out and measured in different laboratories. Chandra asserted that a consistent, standardized, and validated approach to shock tube testing that is capable of producing conventional weapon–level effects in the 10 to 60 psi range is needed to replicate field conditions and facilitate comparisons of findings across different studies and laboratories. He has patented such a candidate approach.

Chandra also noted that while shock tubes are relatively simple to construct and use, they have disadvantages:

- They may not produce an adequate shock/primary blast load.
- They may poorly replicate field conditions.

He warned that one must look at the relationship between static and dynamic pressures and not assume that there is a shock wave. For example, generating a Friedlander wave does not guarantee a shock wave.

Chandra's team, using their shock tube model, has found that with five blasts of less than 5 psi and 3–7 milliseconds of overpressure duration, there are changes to the BBB, indicating biomedical loading. However, the team did not observe these changes in a single blast. Additional tests were insignificant for observations of clotting in the blood serum, sleep studies, and anxiety response. These findings suggest that, among these rodents, a relatively low-level repeated primary blast has potentially important effects on BBB permeability. He speculated that blast overpressure intensity and duration, relative body orientation, animal species, and protective devices are likely to affect these findings.

Predictive Injury Risk Curves for Blast-Related TBI Through Computational Modeling of Multiparametric Empirical Data

Tim Walilko (Applied Research Associates, Inc.) presented results from the Blast Load Assessment Sense and Test study. Using computer models and live miniature pigs, the team sought to inform sensor-based standdown guidelines for blast-exposed service members. Walilko and colleagues hypothesized that if existing neurological studies could be augmented with experimental modeling, then a predictive algorithm could be calculated for blast-induced neurological changes in humans. The team leveraged four human studies, breacher studies, and three large animal studies. In addition, they looked for a single exposure threshold in an animal model and whether multiple subthreshold exposures produced an effect similar to a single threshold exposure. The three animal study arms were (1) single blast of 20–80 psi (blue line), (2) three blasts of 49 psi in a single day (orange line), and (3) one blast of 28 or 51 psi on three consecutive days (red and purple lines, respectively). The results are plotted in Figure 5.10, and

MRI/DTI analysis found that the three subthreshold exposures had an effect equivalent to the single high-intensity blast.

Figure 5.10. Accumulative Effect of Primary Blast Exposure Based on MRI/DTI Findings

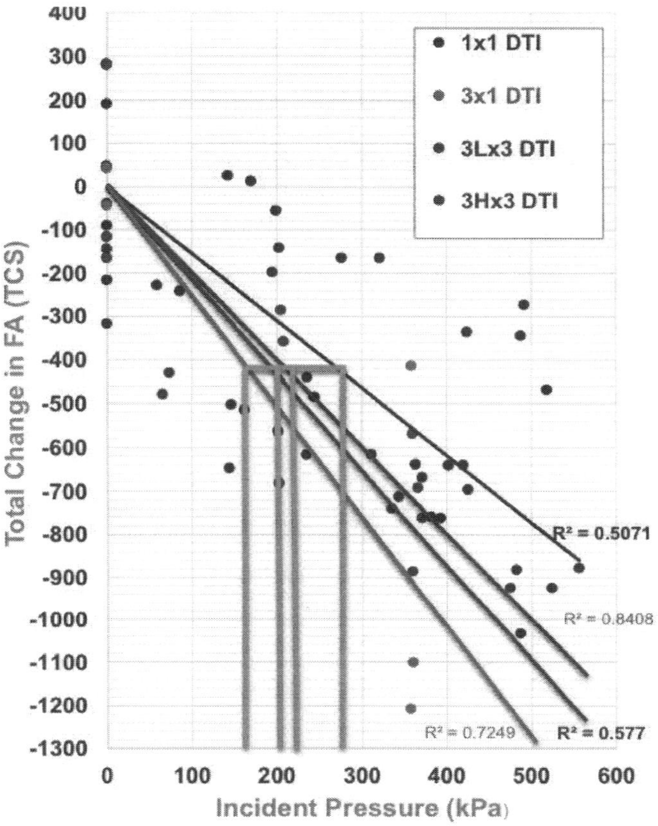

SOURCE: Walilko, 2018.
NOTE: FA = fractional anisotropy. TCS = transcranial current brain stimulation.

Additional analyses included biomechanical algorithms to determine whether blast energy transmitted through the skull has a similar effect on pigs and humans; immunohistochemical analysis using Flouro-Jade, an anionic fluorochrome that selectively stains degenerating neurons; and behavioral assessment of exposed pigs using the Human Approach Test. That test observes changes in behaviors related to appetite versus avoidance with a limited experimental timeline. Results from the combined studies can be used to develop sensor guidelines to monitor service members in training and in combat.

Building Translational Bridges Linking Animal Blast Model Pathology to Neuroimaging and Neuropathology Findings in Veterans with Blast-Related mTBI

David Cook (VA Puget Sound and University of Washington) explained that there is a growing body of evidence that repeated mTBI injuries can result in neurodegenerative diseases. Cook and colleagues used a transgenic animal model to look at the microvascular system with real-time in vivo imaging. They asserted that this is a suitable animal model to study the mechanisms by which repeated low-level blast can cause behavioral and neurological dysfunction. Low-level blasts produced highly localized microdomains of transient BBB disintegration in the posterior cerebellum. In addition, exposed veterans' Purkinje cells degenerated in a similar pattern to those of retired boxers. The study of human brain stems found that blast exposure increases in vivo phasic dopamine release in the nucleus accumbens. This can affect the reward and reinforcement system of the brain known to modulate risk seeking, disinhibition, and addictive behaviors.

An Enhanced Human Surrogate Head Model for Evaluating Blast Injury Mitigation Strategies

Catherine Carneal (Johns Hopkins University Applied Physics Laboratory) shared an enhanced human surrogate head model (Figure 5.11) for evaluating blast mitigation strategies. Human surrogate head models are used to address gaps in understanding of blast-induced brain injury. They characterize the mechanics of blast wave interactions with the head and help researchers study the efficacy of protective equipment to mitigate the biomechanical effects of blast exposures, such as pressure dose and intracranial pressure. Earlier models were similar to those used in automotive testing (e.g., crash-test dummies) and lacked an ability to test helmets, eye protection, or other PPE.

Figure 5.11. Basic Human Surrogate Head Model

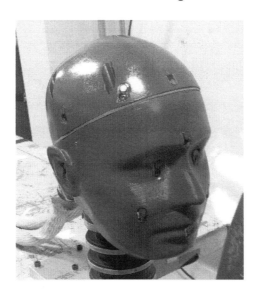

SOURCE: Carneal, 2018.

Live-fire tests were more powerful than those that induced mTBI, but trends can be drawn to learn about directionality, the motion of the head, acceleration, and the effect of PPE.

Changes in Monoamine and Galanin Systems Following Single and Repeated Exposure to Primary Blast

Mårten Risling (Karolinska Institutet) studied whether there are changes in monoamine and galanin in brain tissue following single and repeated exposure to primary blast. There are four components of blast TBI: primary blast wave, focal impact, rotational acceleration, and heat, gas, and electromagnetic pulse (EMP) emission (Figure 5.12).

Figure 5.12. Components of Blast TBIs

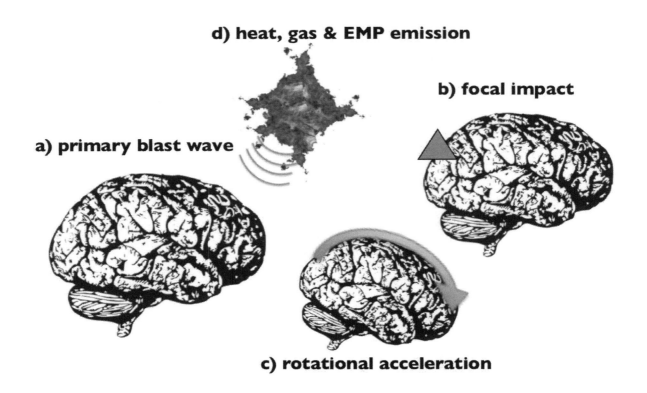

SOURCE: Risling, 2018.

Risling and colleagues examined different blast mechanisms and models to study varying effects. Similar to Elder's experiments, blast tube recordings of pressure waves using mice found considerable overlap between mild blast TBI and PTSD symptoms. Pathological study of exposed mice found increased levels of the enzyme norodine, which protects against oxidative stress. No effect was found on the dorsal raphe nucleus, which produces serotonin in the brain, nor was there any cumulative effect on galanin messenger RNA levels. Galanin is an amino acid neuropeptide that is known to inhibit the neuronal firing and release of neurotransmitters and is implicated in inflammation and mood disorders. The blast tube experiments, visualized in Figure 5.13, provide a foundation for future research. New experiments should include rotational injury to see whether there are similar results without primary blast and to look at how findings can be translated to humans.

Figure 5.13. Blast Tube Experiments with Mice

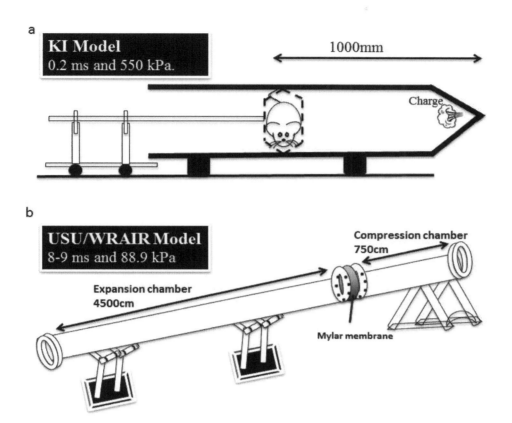

SOURCE: Risling, 2018.
NOTE: KI = knock-in, referring to genetically altered mice. USU/WRAIR = Uniformed Services University/Walter Reed Army Institute of Research.

6. Working Group Summary

On the second and third days of the meeting, participants divided into five working groups, with an expert panelist chairing each. Working group members discussed and addressed four questions (listed below) with the aid of a group-nominated discussion facilitator and note-taker. Groups centered their discussion around perceived gaps, implications, and opportunities. On the fourth day, the expert panel met with the RAND team to combine, collate, and summarize working group responses. This chapter captures insights from that process.

The general consensus among the working groups and expert panelists was that there are more questions than evidence-based answers related to the neurologic effects of repeated, low-level military occupational blast exposure.

Question 1. What Is Known About the Occurrence of Repeated Low-Level Blast Exposure Incurred During Military Service?

While there is little doubt that repeated military occupational blast exposure occurs, there is strikingly little empirical knowledge of its frequency and the military contexts and occupational specialties at greatest risk. A critical obstacle to characterizing the epidemiology of military occupational blast is the lack of an operationalized, consensus definition. Therefore, definition development is a top priority. *Military occupational blast exposure* was predefined for the purpose of the SoSM as exposure to a sudden, explosive pressure change due to heavy munitions firing or activities such as breaching.

An optimal definition will be one based on research that identifies aspects of military occupational blast exposure related to neurological and general health risk, in both short- and long-terms following exposure. Examples within a single exposure may include peak, rise time, duration, impulse, frequency, and sequencing of pressure change and shape of the pressure wave (waveform). Other factors likely to prove important to blast exposure assessment are the number of past exposures, including such characteristics as exposure density (number of exposures per unit of time); residual auditory, optical, and postconcussive effects resulting from blast exposure; and the severity, recency, and mechanisms of past exposures. Aspects of military or social context should also be considered (e.g., firing munitions versus taking fire).

Knowing the contributions of key exposure components to various neurological and general health outcomes may lead to an index score that could be used to estimate individual exposures. Such a score could be based on in-depth measurements of research samples for the purpose of generalizing to blast-exposed military personnel or units. This score may also be used to estimate risk for research purposes (e.g., determining whether there are exposure thresholds, identifying the impact of training exposure on service member health) and then applied for analysis and used for decisionmaking with regard to combat readiness and health risk. This may eventually help determine safe levels of cumulative blast exposure and blast frequency.

To assess the occurrence of exposure, more information is needed about the use of various munition systems in military training and in deployed environments. Cataloging the common blast loads associated with various munition types and military training experiences in a database may help characterize and document data on exposure to low-level blasts, munition types, and environmental occupational context. A consolidated library of the blast characteristics of various munitions could be shared across services and used to map weapon systems, pressure profiles, blast environments, and loading patterns to various neurological and general health risks. This information may also be valuable for medical recordkeeping, as it may aid clinical decisionmaking and research assessments of the long-term consequences of blast exposure.

Question 2. What Is the Scientific Evidence Related to the Potential Neurological Health Effects?

There is little published evidence linking repeated low-level MOBs to neurological injury, symptoms, deficits, and performance effects. Experimental evidence in animals and small observational studies of individuals in certain high-risk occupations (e.g., breachers) suggests that transient cognitive changes can occur. Changes in working memory observed after sleep deprivation or extended exercise are comparable in severity to those seen after repeated low-level blast exposures. There is no evidence of long-term symptoms or deficits related to blast exposure among military personnel, but data collection is needed to look into this risk. Animal studies have generally used rodent models that may not translate easily to humans, and it is not clear that concussive "shock tube" models can be used to investigate the impact of subconcussive blast sustained by military personnel.

Integrating ("embedding") researchers into training and deployed units may improve data collection and the applicability of these data for studies addressing blast effects on service members, such as trainers. A similar approach has been used to collect data on cohorts of athletes. Munitions range instructors represent a unique population of research interest. These instructors are the most likely to be exposed to repeated, low-level blasts, placing them at a potentially higher risk for neurological impairments. Efforts to longitudinally assess cumulative exposure to blast and threshold exposure effects on neurological and general health outcomes should involve baseline and follow-up neuropsychologic, neuroimaging (e.g., diffusion tensor imaging), and physiologic measures. Of interest are factors associated with variation in outcomes, including resilience, susceptibility, and the priming effects of past blast and other exposures. Biomarkers, including genetic factors, may eventually help explain this variation, but, at present, this idea remains speculative.

Question 3. What Are Promising Strategies for Preventing Neurological Damage?

Given the paucity of definitive evidence pertaining to the onset, persistence, and effective treatment of neurological effects after repeated, low-level occupational blast exposure, more emphasis should be placed on improving compliance with currently used protective measures and related policies aimed at reducing general blast exposure. Testing of new methods aiming to mitigate exposure should assess for potential adverse effects on readiness and health, as well as effectiveness against low-level blast exposure.

Policy efforts should focus immediately on current DoD and military service policies, directives, instructions, standards, and safety guidelines. For example, the technical manuals for weapon systems include weapon-specific, health-based standards that mandate the use of single or double hearing-protection devices to help prevent auditory injury; that limit the number of rounds fired per day; or that place restrictions on firing from certain positions, such as from enclosures or from the prone position to protect against primary blast injuries to internal organs (e.g., the lungs). Ensuring awareness of and compliance with policies and guidelines pertaining to PPE and measures using a functional solutions analysis approach is an essential preventive step.

Intermediate- and long-term research aims should include well-designed evaluations of improved compliance with PPE guidance, organizational policies and practices, and evidence on the intended and unintended impacts on readiness and health. Potentially promising innovations include low-level blast-canceling devices and munition systems that reduce the potential for human exposure and risk (e.g., robotics, drones).

Question 4. What Are Promising Indicators for Early Detection of Potential Neurological Consequences?

There are numerous potentially applicable indicators available or in development. The utility of any of these indicators has yet to be established for low-level, military occupational blast exposure. Selection of a given indicator will depend on the outcome of specific interest, and the theoretical and empirical evidence in support of its use. The priority should be to select indicators for study that are feasible to use in military contexts (e.g., those that do not inhibit service member performance), address theoretical or operational measurement domains of interest, and are demonstrably reliable and valid for the purpose intended. To adapt these and newer indicators, unit-based ("embedded") research collaborations involving bioengineers, biomedical specialists, device developers, and end users should be pursued.

These potential indicators are as follows:
- biofluid biomarkers (e.g., blood, saliva, urine, sweat, breath, cerebrospinal fluid)
- neuroimaging
- ocular-motor testing
- neuromotor variability

- gene expression changes
- audiologic temporary threshold shift (e.g., central auditory screening tool)
- vestibular changes
- cognitive working memory
- quantitative electroencephalogram
- protein assays, including neuroendocrine
- speech annoyance tool
- optical coherence tomography
- brief, automated neuropsychological assessments
- psychological assessment tool for behavior and mood
- TBI/concussion markers (e.g., brain injury survey questionnaire [BISQ] form, concussion subtyping [Ghajar], acute concussion evaluations [DANA, MACE])
- general and blast specific symptomology at baseline
- blast-specific questionnaire for self-reported symptoms linked to environment
- autonomic changes through heart rate variability
- audiometric measures for peripheral and central
- activity and sleep monitoring using wearable actigraphy
- vestibular and ocular-motor (e.g., eye tracking, VOMS, balance)
- working memory and impulse control cognitive tests (e.g., go/no-go task).

7. State-of-the-Science Meeting Recommendations

The following recommendations were compiled by the SoSM expert panel for the Secretary of Defense and senior military leaders.

Recommendation 1

Enforce DoD policies and standards related to low-level MOB exposure. Review the implementation of current policies and standards, and monitor compliance. Educate those responsible for applying policies and standards, and rigorously evaluate efforts to improve compliance with them.

Recommendation 2

Develop a portfolio of high-quality studies assessing occurrences of repeated, low-level occupational blast injury. These studies should (1) characterize how often service members are exposed to low-level blasts; (2) define the context (e.g., training, deployed) and environmental conditions associated with exposures; (3) assess and disseminate primary blast parameters for all unclassified weapon systems; and (4) assess the potential for exposure among high-risk occupational specialties, such as breachers, artillery personnel, grenade range trainers, and other regular users of heavy weaponry.

Recommendation 3

Prepare and plan, in response to recent congressional legislation, for a large-scale population-based longitudinal study of military personnel with long-term follow-up to assess the prevalence and severity of neurological and general health outcomes after repeated, low-level MOBs. The study should include measures of low-level blast exposure over time and assess the linkages between these exposures (including key exposure characteristics) and neurological and general health outcomes to determine whether repeated, low-level blast exposure increases risk. Contributors to the study should include military operations experts, bioengineers, physiologists, neuroscientists, neuropsychologists, epidemiologists, and clinician-researchers. The study should oversample breachers and other occupations that require working in settings with high expected risk of exposure to heavy weaponry or other sources of repeated, low-level blasts (see Recommendation 2). Study sampling should take into account potential variations in outcomes by gender, age, rank, and cumulative history of blast exposures, as well as service members' medical, military, and psychiatric histories. Post-mortem storage of brain tissue may eventually allow researchers to link longitudinal exposure data to structural brain outcomes.

Recommendation 4

Transition the focus of animal studies of repeated, low-level blast exposure from rodents to larger animals, including nonhuman primate models. Animal studies should be guided by suspected symptoms and deficits related to blast exposure, designed to identify the mechanisms that underlie clinical findings, and test approximate exposure conditions observed in human research. These efforts will maximize the translation of animal findings to humans. Animal models remain important because they allow carefully controlled research that addresses confounding variables and allow for the experimental manipulation of exposure types and context in ways that are unfeasible or unethical in human studies. Laboratories completing these studies should coordinate efforts to ensure that exposure paradigms are consistent across sites so that results from different laboratories can be more easily compared. Shock-tube models used for studying the effects of concussive blasts do not necessarily model subconcussive blasts. Animal experiments in real-world military exposure contexts may prove informative in some instances. Similar to the proposed human studies, animal studies should control for variation by gender and age.

Recommendation 5

Studies that examine the possible neurologic and general health effects of low-level blast exposure indicators should align with current military exposure assessment tools and protective practices and devices when this is feasible while adhering to the objectives of the study. This strategy is more likely to result in incremental improvements to current military practices.

Recommendation 6

Catalogue, map, and make available to researchers, safety programs, and military end users unclassified weapon system–specific information, including blast pressure profiles and service member–specific load profiles. Build a consolidated library of such exposures for key military contexts, such as breaching, military policing, and deployment, and for training-specific uses of heavy weaponry (e.g., artillery, grenade-range training).

Recommendation 7

Design policies and increase opportunities for the use of embedded research scientists from key disciplines (e.g., military end users, bioengineers, biomedical researchers, neuroscientists, neuropsychologists, epidemiologists, clinician-researchers) within units during training and in deployed contexts. This will ensure the military relevance, timeliness, and continuity of emerging studies addressing real-world military questions and contexts and will improve the operational usefulness and ecological validity of novel preventive interventions.

Appendix A. Planning Committee

This meeting was made possible thanks to the guidance, planning, and insights of the members of the SoSM planning committee, whose members are listed here.

Stephen Ahlers
Naval Medical Research Center

Pat Bellgowan
National Institutes of Health

MAJ Walter Carr
Center for Military Psychiatry and Neuroscience, Walter Reed Army Institute of Research

Namas Chandra
New Jersey Institute of Technology

David Cooper
Vision Center of Excellence T2

CAPT Scott Cota
U.S. Special Operations Command

Thomas DeGraba
National Intrepid Center of Excellence

Stefan Duma
Virginia Tech University

Charles Engel
RAND Corporation

Louis French
National Intrepid Center of Excellence, Walter Reed National Military Medical Center

Ramona Hicks
OneMind

COL Sidney Hinds
DoD Blast Injury Research Program Coordinating Office

Stuart Hoffman
Office of Research and Development, U.S. Department of Veterans Affairs

Christopher Hoppel
Army Research Laboratory

Grace Hwang
Johns Hopkins University Applied Physics Laboratory

Todd Jaszewski
Joint Program Committee–5, Army Medical Research and Materiel Command

Vassilis Koliatsos
Johns Hopkins University School of Medicine

Theresa (Tracie) Lattimore
Office of the Surgeon General, Army Medical Command

Donald Marion
Defense and Veterans Brain Injury Center

COL(R) Robert Mazzoli
DoD-VA Vision Center of Excellence

COL Dennis McGurk
Joint Program Committee–5, Army Medical
Research and Materiel Command

Anthony Pacifico
Congressionally Directed Medical Research
Programs, Army Medical Research and
Materiel Command

James B. Petro
Office of the Assistant Secretary of Defense
for Research and Engineering

Bryan Pfister
New Jersey Institute of Technology

CDR Randy Reese
Navy Bureau of Medicine and Surgery

Tyler Rooks
Army Aeromedical Research Laboratory

Deborah Shear
Walter Reed Army Institute of Research

Matthew Sherer
Joint Program Committee–5, Army Medical
Research and Materiel Command

Richard Shoge
Joint Program Committee–5, Army Medical
Research and Materiel Command

Victoria Tepe
DoD-VA Hearing Center of Excellence

CAPT Penny Walter
DoD-VA Vision Center of Excellence

Keith Whitaker
Army Research Laboratory

Julie Wilberding
Uniformed Services University, Center for
Neuroscience and Regenerative Medicine

Appendix B. Meeting Agenda

Monday, March 12, 2018

Time	Schedule	Presenter
8:00	Registration opens	
8:30	*Welcome from the Department of Defense Blast Injury Research Program Coordinating Office*	Michael Leggieri Director, DoD Blast Injury Research Program Coordinating Office
8:40	*General Meeting Overview*	Charles Engel, MD, MPH RAND Senior Scientist and Principal Investigator, Seventh State-of-the-Science Meeting
8:45	**Keynote Speaker**	**MG Malcolm Frost, Army Commanding General, Center for Initial Military Training, Army Training and Doctrine Command**
9:25	***Discussion Panel: Strategy—DoD Policy and Requirements***	

Panel Moderator: COL Dennis McGurk, PhD, Director, Military Operational Medicine Research Program, Army Medical Research and Materiel Command

MG Malcolm Frost, Commanding General, Center for Initial Military Training, Army Training and Doctrine Command

Elizabeth Fudge, MSN, MPH, Executive Officer, Office of the Assistant Secretary of Defense for Health Affairs, Health Readiness Policy and Oversight

Timothy Kluchinsky, Jr., DrPH, MSPH, Chief, Health Hazard Assessment Division, Army Public Health Center

James Zheng, PhD, Chief Scientist, Project Manager Soldier Protection and Individual Equipment, Army Program Executive Office–Soldier

Time	Schedule	Presenter
10:45	**AM BREAK**	
11:00	***Summary of RAND Literature Review***	Charles Engel, MD, MPH Senior Scientist, RAND Corporation
11:45	**LUNCH and POSTER SET-UP**	

1:15	*Discussion Panel: State of Current Research and Solutions*

Panel Moderator: Grace Hwang, PhD, Program Manager, Neurological Health and Human Performance Program, Research and Exploratory Development Department, Johns Hopkins University Applied Physics Laboratory

MAJ Walter Carr, PhD, Center for Military Psychiatry and Neuroscience, Walter Reed Army Institute of Research

Ibolja Cernak, MD, PhD, STARR-C (Stress, Trauma and Resilience Research Consulting) LLC

Vassilis Koliatsos, MD, Professor of Pathology and Neurology, Johns Hopkins University School of Medicine

James Stone, MD, PhD, Vice Chair of Research, Department of Radiology and Medical Imaging, University of Virginia

Jonathan Touryan, PhD, Research Scientist, Center for Adaptive Soldier Technologies, Human Research and Engineering Directorate, Army Research Laboratory

2:45	**PM BREAK**

3:00	*Scientific Session 1: Direct Measurements and Prospective Assessment*	**Moderator:** Charles Engel, MD, MPH Senior Scientist, RAND Corporation

	Understanding Potential Neurological Consequences and Mechanisms of Repeated Blast Exposure	CDR Josh Duckworth, MD
	Profiling of Blast-Overpressure Effects on the Human Brain in Breacher Training	Jia Lu, MD, PhD
	Quantifying Occupational Blast Exposure During Military and Law Enforcement Training	Gary Kamimori, PhD
	Receiving a Multiple Peak Blast Dose in a Single Complex Blast Event	Jean-Philippe Dionne, PhD
	Q&A Panel	

4:45	**Adjourn**

Tuesday, March 13, 2018

Time	Schedule	Presenter
8:00	**Welcome** ***Scientific Session 2: Inferred Occupational Exposure***	**Moderator:** Charles Engel, MD, MPH Senior Scientist, RAND Corporation
	Suicide in Combatants with Extensive Blast Exposure: Strictly a Mental Health Issue or Evidence of Underlying Structural Brain Lesions?	Daniel Perl, MD
	Impaired Stress Coping and Cognitive Function Caused by Blast Exposure	Ibolja Cernak, MD, PhD
	Occupational Risk Moderates the Relationship Between Major Blast Exposure and Traumatic Brain Injury	Jennifer Belding, PhD
	Epidemiologic Study of Occupational Blast Exposure and Subsequent Diagnoses	MAJ Walter Carr, PhD
	Q&A Panel	
9:45	**AM BREAK**	
10:00	***Scientific Session 3: Animal Studies and Their Translation***	**Moderator:** Charles Engel, MD, MPH Senior Scientist, RAND Corporation
	Blast-induced "PTSD": Evidence from an Animal Model	Greg Elder, MD
	The Dynamics of Structural Changes After Repeated Mild Blast TBI: Acute Pathologies and Lasting Consequences	Denes Agoston, MD, PhD
	Neuronal Response to Multiple Shock Tube Overpressure Exposures	Thomas O'Shaughnessy, PhD
	Blood-Brain Barrier Permeability Is a Sensitive Neurological Marker for Single and Repeated Occupational Low-Level Blast Exposures in a Rodent Model	Namas Chandra, PhD
	Q&A Panel	
11:30	**LUNCH and POSTER SESSION**	
12:30	***Scientific Session 4: Prevention and Biomarkers***	**Moderator:** Charles Engel, MD, MPH Senior Scientist, RAND Corporation
	Predictive Injury Risk Curves for Blast-Related TBI Through Computational Modeling of Multi-Parametric Empirical Data	Tim Walilko, PhD

	Building Translational Bridges Linking Animal Blast Model Pathology to Neuroimaging and Neuropathology Findings in Veterans with Blast-Related mTBI	David Cook, PhD
	An Enhanced Human Surrogate Head Model for Evaluating Blast Injury Mitigation Strategies	Catherine Carneal
	Changes in Monoamine and Galanin Systems Following Single and Repeated Exposure to Primary Blast	Mårten Risling, MD, PhD
	Q&A Panel	
2:00	*Introduction to the Working Groups*	**Moderator:** Charles Engel, MD, MPH Senior Scientist, RAND Corporation
2:15	**PM BREAK**	
2:45	*Working Groups Begin**	Chaired by the expert panelists
5:30	*Adjourn Directly from Working Groups*	

Breaks determined by members of each working group.

Wednesday, March 14, 2018

Time	Schedule	Presenter
8:00	*Working Groups, Continued**	Chaired by the expert panelists
11:30	**LUNCH and POSTER SESSION**	
12:30	*Working Groups, Continued**	Chaired by the expert panelists
2:30	**PM BREAK**	
2:30	*Working Group Reports*	Working group representatives
4:30	*Closing Remarks and Adjourn*	Michael Leggieri Director, Blast Injury Research Program Coordinating Office

Breaks determined by members of each working group.

Appendix C. Keynote Speaker Biography

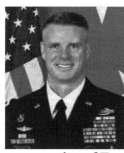

MG Malcolm B. Frost

MG Malcolm B. Frost is the commanding general for the Army Center for Initial Military Training, Army Training and Doctrine Command, and is responsible for annually transforming 120,000 civilian volunteers into soldiers who are physically ready, grounded in Army values, competent in their skills, and able to contribute as leaders and team members upon arrival at their first Army unit of assignment. He also serves as the senior mission commander of Fort Eustis as part of Joint Base Langley-Eustis, Virginia.

Prior to his arrival at Fort Eustis, MG Frost served as the Army Chief of Public Affairs and was responsible for all communication involving the Army; charged with formulating communication and public affairs strategies, plans and policies; and served as the senior adviser to the Secretary of the Army and Chief of Staff of the Army on communication matters.

MG Frost served in infantry leadership and staff positions as a company-grade officer while assigned to the 1st Battalion, 8th Infantry, 4th Infantry Division, at Fort Carson, Colorado; 3rd Battalion, 325th Infantry Airborne Battalion in Vicenza, Italy; and the 3rd Infantry (The Old Guard) at Fort Myer, Virginia. His service in Italy included company command in Bosnia-Herzegovina in 1995 during Operation Joint Endeavor. In 1996–1998, he served as aide-de-camp to the 33rd Chief of Staff of the Army. He later served in the 82nd Airborne Division at Fort Bragg, North Carolina, including as the 1st Brigade's operations officer in 2002–2003 during Operation Enduring Freedom in Afghanistan.

MG Frost served in Hawaii in 2003–2005 as the 25th Infantry Division operations officer and chief of staff for the 25th Infantry Division Rear. He then commanded the 2nd Battalion, 5th Infantry Regiment, and, later, the 3rd Squadron, 4th Cavalry Regiment, 3rd Infantry Brigade Combat Team, 25th Infantry Division, which included deployment to Iraq in 2006–2007 during the Operation Iraqi Freedom surge.

MG Frost returned to Hawaii in 2009 after attending the Army War College. He commanded the 2nd Stryker Brigade Combat Team, 25th Infantry Division, at Schofield Barracks. This assignment coincided with the unit's deployment to Iraq in 2010–2011, where it served as an advise-and-assist brigade in support of Operations Iraqi Freedom and New Dawn. MG Frost later served for a year at Fort Shafter as the Army Pacific Deputy Chief of Staff for Operations, G3/5/7/9.

MG Frost received his commission in the infantry after graduating from the United States Military Academy at West Point, New York, in 1988. He holds master's degrees in human resources development from Webster University and national security studies from the Army War College.

His awards and decorations include the Distinguished Service Medal, Defense Superior Service Medal, Legion of Merit (third award), Bronze Star Medal (third award), Meritorious Service Medal (sixth award), Air Medal, Army Commendation Medal (sixth award, one for valor), Army Achievement Medal (second award), Ranger Tab, Master Parachutist Badge, Combat Infantryman's Badge, Expert Infantryman's Badge, Department of State Meritorious Honor Award, Joint Chiefs of Staff Identification Badge, and the Department of the Army Staff Identification Badge.

Appendix D. Discussion Panel Biographies

This year, the SoSM included two plenary session discussion panels. Each panel was a moderated discussion involving knowledgeable researchers, military leaders, policymakers, and clinicians. The discussion panels are designed to foster dialogue with the audience and among the panelists.

MG Malcolm B. Frost
See keynote speaker biography in Appendix C.

LTC James R. McKnight, DrPH

LTC James McKnight has a BS in microbiology from Northern Illinois University, a master's degree in infectious disease epidemiology from the University of Iowa, and a doctor of public health degree in global health practice from the University of South Florida. LTC McKnight was direct commissioned a first lieutenant in the Medical Service Corps, Army Medical Department.

His initial assignment was to Landstuhl, Germany, where he served as the assistant chief of the Environmental Health Division, Department of Preventive Medicine, Landstuhl Regional Medical Center. After four and a half years in Germany, LTC McKnight was assigned to Group Support Company, Group Support Battalion, 3rd Special Forces Group (Airborne), Fort Bragg, North Carolina, where he served as the group preventive medicine officer, group support company executive officer, rear detachment commander, and service support commander (while deployed). During his time with 3rd Special Forces Group (Airborne), LTC McKnight deployed to Afghanistan twice in support of Operation Enduring Freedom. LTC McKnight's next assignment was to serve as chief of environmental health, Preventive Medicine Services, Blanchfield Army Community Hospital, Fort Campbell, Kentucky. He also served as vice president of the Junior Officer Council.

After two years at Fort Campbell, LTC McKnight was selected for Long Term Healthcare Education Training to pursue his doctorate degree. While pursuing his DrPH, LTC McKnight was assigned to U.S. Central Command as a follow-on utilization tour, where he worked as a force health protection officer. LTC McKnight currently works as an environmental science engineering officer and is acting deputy director for the Military Operational Medicine Research Program at Fort Detrick, Maryland.

His military education includes Airborne School, Rigger School, Army Medical Department Officer's Basic Course, Captain's Career Course, Intermediate Level Education/Command and General Staff College, Industrial Hygiene Course, Principles of Preventive Medicine Course, Hazardous Waste Operations and Emergency Course,

Environmental Quality Officer's Course, Medical Management of Biological and Chemical Casualties Course, and Transport of Biomedical Material Course.

His awards and decorations include the Bronze Star, the Defense Meritorious Service Medal, the Meritorious Service Medal (third award), the Joint Service Commendation Award, the Army Achievement Medal (third award), the Meritorious Unit Citation, the Joint Meritorious Unit Award (third award), the Army Superior Unit Award, the National Defense Service Medal (second award), the NATO Medal, the Afghanistan Campaign Medal (second award), the Global War of Terrorism Service Medal, the Army Service Ribbon, the Overseas Service Ribbon, the Royal Netherlands Parachutist Badge, the German Parachutist Badge, the Parachute Rigger Badge, and Parachutist Badge.

MAJ Walter Carr, PhD

MAJ Carr holds a doctorate in experimental psychology and has a ten-year line of research related to the neurological effects of repeated MOB exposure. A key target of his program is to elucidate the consequences of chronic exposure to blast and/or concussive events, including contributions to technical requirements and methodologies for wearable environmental sensor technologies in selected Department of Defense training. He has led and been engaged with an active series of human subject protocols, gathering data and refining techniques for the study of neurocognitive and neurophysiological effects following blast exposure. Methods and measures to evaluate such exposures and consequent effects are still being improved and validated, as is an association with individual difference factors. This area of responsibility includes epidemiology, basic science, and prospective field-based studies and is directly aligned with priority topics in military medicine. MAJ Carr currently serves as a branch chief in the Center for Military Psychiatry and Neuroscience at the Walter Reed Army Institute of Research.

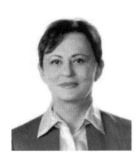

Dr. Ibolja Cernak, MD, PhD

Dr. Cernak is president of STARR-C (Stress, Trauma and Resilience Research Consulting) LLC. She has broad multidisciplinary expertise, including an MD, an MS in biomedical engineering, an MS in homeland security (public health preparedness), and a PhD in pathophysiology and neuroscience. Previously, Dr. Cernak was a medical director and principal professional staff (tenured professor equivalent) at the Johns Hopkins University Applied Physics Laboratory; associate professor of neuroscience at Georgetown University, visiting professor at James Cook University in Townsville, Queensland, Australia; visiting professor at the 3rd Military Medical University, Chongqing, People's Republic of China; and professor of clinical pathophysiology in Belgrade, Serbia (formerly Yugoslavia).

With more than 30 years of experience, Dr. Cernak is world-renowned for her clinical and experimental research on blast injuries, including blast-induced neurotrauma.

Her research also includes traumatic brain injury of various etiologies focusing on the mechanisms of trauma-induced long-term neurological and mental health impairments, stress response and resilience to occupational stress, and predictors of injury and increased susceptibility to illnesses/injuries in military and first responder populations.

Dr. Cernak has published more than 200 research articles in international refereed journals, served as a keynote or invited speaker at more than 300 professional meetings, and filed three patents. She is a member of several professional bodies, including three subject committees of the Institute of Medicine, on the long-term consequences of traumatic brain injury in veterans, on soldiers' readjustment problems, and on the long-term consequences of blast exposure, as well as the NATO Human Force and Medicine task groups focusing on blast and other military injuries.

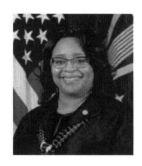

Ms. Elizabeth R. Fudge, MSN, MPH

Ms. Elizabeth Fudge is the executive officer, Office of the Assistant Secretary of Defense for Health Affairs, Health Readiness Policy and Oversight (HRP&O). In this capacity, she serves as principal adviser, managing overall planning and engagement activities and tasks of the policy directors and staff. Among her many areas of oversight responsibility for medical readiness are medical countermeasures, medical logistics, preparedness, preventive health, operational medicine, global health engagement, research and development, and research regulatory oversight. Another major responsibility is overseeing HRP&O interaction with the military departments, Congress, and various executive branch agencies and ensuring that health care programs and policies correspond to department goals.

Ms. Fudge's has a BS in nursing from the University of Michigan, an MPH from Tulane University, and a master of science in nursing from Emory University. While serving in the Army she attended the Army Command and General Staff College. Her advanced practice credentials include certification as a family nurse practitioner.

Prior to her current assignment, which she assumed in January 2017, Ms. Fudge served in the Defense Health Agency, Healthcare Operations, Readiness Division, as branch chief for operational medicine from 2012 to 2014. Her responsibilities included leading teams in developing and updating DoD policies for traumatic brain injury, DoD use of computerized neurocognitive assessments, combat casualty care and the Joint Trauma System, medical readiness training, and combat pre-hospital documentation and patient movement. After retiring from the Army in 2006 with 20 years of service, Ms. Fudge began her federal civilian career supporting the Military Health System as a senior health policy analyst in the Office of the Assistant Secretary of Defense for Health Affairs and the Force Health Protection and Readiness programs.

Ms. Fudge was briefly a staff nurse practitioner at a private practice in Leesburg, Virginia, after serving as director of Army public health and occupational health nursing and assistant director of nursing at Walter Reed Army Medical Center (2004–2006). In 2002–2003 she served as director of preventive medicine services at Soto Cano Air Base, Honduras, and was stationed at McDonald Army Community Hospital at Fort Eustis, Virginia, as nursing director of community and occupational health and at Brooke Army Medical Center, Fort Sam Houston, Texas, as a staff family nurse practitioner (1999–2002).

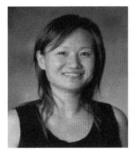

Dr. Grace Hwang, PhD

Grace M. Hwang is a principal investigator at the Johns Hopkins University Applied Physics Laboratory. She holds an MS in civil and environmental engineering from the Massachusetts Institute of Technology and an MS and a PhD in biophysics and structural biology from Brandeis University. Her dissertation research focused on the analysis of human electroencephalography to understand the neural basis of visual and verbal memory, for which she developed novel nonparametric statistical techniques for high-dimensional data for across- and within-subject multifactorial analysis. Presently, she studies noninvasive methods of neurostimulation and imaging with the goal to drive the development of brain-computer interface applications for healthy people and clinical populations. She is developing low-intensity focused ultrasound and applying digital holographic imaging with the goal of producing high spatiotemporal resolution information noninvasively. She has extensive experience in experimental design, computational cognitive neuroscience, biophysics, biosensors, biomarker discovery, and optical spectroscopy and has authored or co-authored more than 25 peer-reviewed publications.

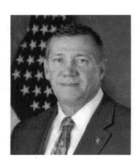

Dr. Timothy Kluchinsky, Jr., DrPH, MSPH

Dr. Kluchinsky is assigned to the Army Public Health Center, Aberdeen Proving Ground, Maryland, where he manages the Health Hazard Assessment Program in support of the materiel acquisition process. He holds a master's degree in basic science from the University of Colorado, and both an MS in public health and a DrPH from the Uniformed Services University.

Dr. Kluchinsky is a retired soldier who began his military career in 1983 as an enlisted infantry TOW anti-tank missile crewman. He reenlisted in the Air Defense Artillery Branch as a Chaparral missile crewman; received an ROTC scholarship to Pacific Lutheran University, Tacoma, Washington; and was commissioned in 1992 as an air defense artillery officer, serving as both a Stinger platoon leader and Bradley Stinger Fighting Vehicle platoon leader. In 1996, after spending more than half his career in combat arms, Dr. Kluchinsky branch-transferred to the Medical Service Corps to serve as an environmental science and engineering officer.

In 2007, he concluded his 24-year military career while serving as an assistant professor at the Uniformed Services University, Department of Preventive Medicine and Biometrics, to reassume the role as manager of the Army Health Hazard Assessment Program, a position he previously held as an officer assigned to the Army Public Health Center.

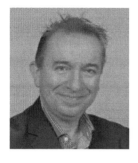

Dr. Vassilis E. Koliatsos, MD

Vassilis E. Koliatsos, MD is a professor of pathology (neuropathology) and neurology and an associate professor of psychiatry and behavioral sciences at the Johns Hopkins University School of Medicine, a clinical professor of psychiatry at the University of Maryland School of Medicine, and the Stulman scholar and director of the neuropsychiatry program at Sheppard and Enoch Pratt Hospital in Baltimore, Maryland. He is a physician-investigator focusing on neural trauma and neurodegeneration. As a clinician, he specializes in the cognitive and behavioral problems of patients with neurodegenerative disease and traumatic brain injury. He has mentored numerous pre- and postdoctoral students and has taught clinical neurosciences and neuropsychiatry to residents in neurology and psychiatry. As a researcher, he focuses on mechanisms of neural injury and repair and regenerative neuroscience at the molecular and systems levels. His current interests regarding TBI are focused on the chronic effects of concussion, particularly the problem of traumatic axonopathy and protein aggregation. He has also pioneered work characterizing the pathological mechanisms of blast TBI in animal models and humans. Dr. Koliatsos has been awarded the Leadership and Excellence in Alzheimer's Disease Award and the Javits Neuroscience Investigator Award, both from the National Institutes of Health.

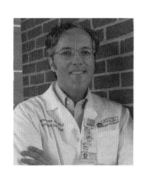

Dr. James Stone, MD, PhD

James R. Stone is an associate professor and vice chair of research in the Department of Radiology and Medical Imaging at the University of Virginia. He is a clinical interventional radiologist with a neuroscience background. His laboratory currently explores questions related to improving the clinical diagnosis of traumatic brain injury (TBI) in both preclinical models and human subjects. Ongoing preclinical work includes the design and investigation of molecular imaging probes for detecting acute and chronic effects of TBI. Probes under investigation include those targeting inflammation, cell death, and altered neurotransmitter receptor activity. He is involved in exploring neurovascular changes in a preclinical blast TBI model. Human subjects efforts have focused on the neuroimaging correlates of repetitive low-level blast exposure in military populations. The goals of this work include determining whether service members in this environment are at risk of developing mild TBI and helping to establish safe stand-off limits for low-level blast exposure. Additionally, Dr. Stone is involved with efforts to build a normative library to support improved population-level research and work toward single-subject assessment of patients with TBI. He is also involved in utilizing machine learning/deep learning approaches for the automated segmentation of imaging findings to diagnose TBI. He is a member of the neuroimaging core laboratory for the Chronic Effects of Neurotrauma Consortium. Dr. Stone's work receives support from the Defense Health Program, Office of Naval Research, and Department of Veterans Affairs. His participation in efforts to establish a normative neuroimaging library receive support from Cohen Veterans Bioscience.

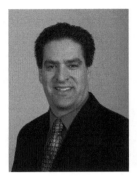

Dr. Jonathan Touryan, PhD

Dr. Jonathan (Jon) Touryan is a research scientist in the Army Research Laboratory's Human Research and Engineering Directorate. He joined the Army Research Laboratory from SAIC (now Leidos) in 2012, where he managed the company's neuroimaging facility and conducted research in human neuroscience for various defense agencies, including the Defense Advanced Research Projects Agency, Army Research Laboratory, and Air Force Research Laboratory. Dr. Touryan received his PhD from the University of California, Berkeley, in 2004, where he studied the neurophysiology of vision. He then conducted postdoctoral research on the neural correlates of visual attention at Yale University School of Medicine. He has published research in a number of leading neuroscience journals and has experience in both human and animal neuroimaging techniques. His most recent work focuses on single-trial classification of brain signals that underlie perception, memory, and cognition. Currently, he works on brain computer interface technology for Army applications and leads the basic science research effort under the Cognition and Neuroergonomics Collaborative Technology Alliance.

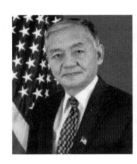

Dr. James Zheng, PhD

Dr. James Zheng is director of the Technical Management Directorate and chief scientist for Project Manager Soldier Protection and Individual Equipment, Army Program Executive Office–Soldier. Dr. Zheng has a bachelor's degree in chemistry and a master's degree in physics from the University of Science and Technology of China. He earned his PhD in physical chemistry from Purdue University. Dr. Zheng holds two patents and has published more than 70 scientific papers.

Dr. Zheng was one of the recipients of the Army's Greatest Invention Award in 2002 for developing a DoD standard body armor system, the Interceptor Multiple Threat Body Armor. He received the Army's Superior Civilian Service Medal in 2008 for "exceptional meritorious and superior technical achievement" for developing the Enhanced Small Arms Protective Insert. In 2009, he received the Program Manager of the Year award from Office of the Secretary of Defense Comparative Testing Office. He is one of the recipients of the 2013 Office of the Secretary of Defense Manufacturing Technology Achievement Award. In 2016, he received the Order of Saint Maurice medal from the National Infantry Association for "representing the highest standards of integrity, moral character, professional competence, and dedication to duty" and his second Superior Civilian Service Medal for "dedication to duty [that] has brought lifesaving personal protective equipment to hundreds of thousands of Infantry Soldiers and saved countless lives."

Appendix E. Poster Abstracts

The following posters were presented at the meeting. The abstracts are presented in alphabetical order by the studies' first author.

Investigating Primary and Reduced Secondary Shock Wave Impact on a Surrogate Head Model

Presenter: Rohan Banton, Army Research Laboratory

Additional authors:
- Thuvan Piehler, Nicole Zander, Randy Mrozek, and Richard Benjamin, Army Research Laboratory
- Josh Duckworth, Uniformed Services University

Repeated blast exposures in military training have led to new concerns about rates of subconcussive and mild TBIs among military personnel. For these personnel, these repeated blast exposures are akin to double-shock exposure. To that end, the current research has investigated the response behavior of a surrogate brain to impact from a primary and reduced secondary shock wave following initiation of a single RDX explosive charge. More specifically, high-speed imaging techniques were utilized to capture the primary and secondary shock wave impact on a surrogate head model following the explosive initiation of 1.7 grams of RDX charge.

The biomechanical response of the surrogate brain to the blast loading from the RDX explosive was assessed for areas of elevated stress and strain. Quantitative pressure loading inside the surrogate head model was determined through the use of strategically placed pressure sensors at a 5-mm depth inside the front, kocher points, and the back of the head. In addition, a finite element model of a human head form filled with biofidelic gel representative of brain tissue was placed in an Eulerian air domain and subjected to simulated blast waves.

The evolution of the primary and secondary shock wave propagation from the site of initiation was fully captured in the numerical simulation and compared well with the high-speed images obtained from the experiment. The simulated primary shock wave impact to the surrogate head was in agreement with the experiment in terms of time of arrival and compressive pressure loading to the skull at 140 microseconds and 300 kPa, respectively. The subsequent secondary shock wave impact to the surrogate head was also captured using the high-speed imaging techniques, and it was also in agreement with the numerical simulation. Unfortunately, visual confirmation of a secondary wave impact was obtained from the imaging technique, and no definitive quantitative results were obtained due to the weak strength of secondary pressure wave and the pressure probe's lack of sensitivity to record at such a weak reading. The results from the numerical simulation also produced a weak secondary pressure wave that attenuated at impact on the surrogate head. The opacity of the skull also prevented the high-speed imaging technique from capturing the intracranial pressure. To overcome this limitation, the numerical model was employed.

The simulated results revealed strong compressive loading in the anterior and posterior regions of the surrogate brain with pressures of 198 and 205 kPa, respectively. Taken together, the numerical and experimental results revealed high compressive and tensile loading, as well as deviatoric stress distribution at the skull/surrogate brain. This indicates the potential for shearing/tearing of brain tissue due to blast loading.

Response of Neurons Following Mechanical Injury in Vitro: Effect of Equal-Biaxial Strain and Strain Rate

Presenter: Ann Mae DiLeonardi, Army Research Laboratory

Additional authors:
- C. Allan Gunnarsson and Tusit Weerasooriya, Army Research Laboratory

TBI occurs when a primary insult causes brain deformation resulting in secondary injury and, ultimately, neuronal degeneration and death. Data suggest that the brain is susceptible to both the strain and strain rate of the insult. To understand how altering the rate of injury affects secondary injury, we cultured primary hippocampal neurons on silicone membranes and stretched them using the cell injury controller II.

First, 2D strain tensor of the membrane, at three different pressures (23, 47, and 63 psi) and three different times to peak (25, 50, and 75 microseconds), was measured using digital image correlation. Strains increased as either pressure or time to peak increased. Maximum principle strain rates were also obtained during the rising part of the strain waveform. Using these strain rates and interpolating between these measurements, maximum principle strain rates were obtained for each pressure and time to peak used in our experiments. Hippocampi were harvested from day E18 rat embryos, cultured, and subjected to a biaxial stretch of 10-mm peak deformation at three different rates ten to 12 days in vitro. Cells from the center region of the membrane where radial and tangential strains were approximately equal (equal-biaxial with negligible shear) were used for analysis of their response after biaxial stretch. Structural damage to neurons was quantified using immunocytochemistry of microtubule-associated protein 2, and functional damage is being evaluated using live cell imaging to visualize changes to cellular transport.

Tauroursodeoxycholic Acid and Sodium Phenylbutyrate for Treatment of Traumatic Brain Injury

Presenter: Afshin Divani, Department of Neurology, University of Minnesota

Additional authors:
- Cecilia M. P. Rodrigues, Research Institute for Medicines (iMed.ULisboa), Faculty of Pharmacy, University of Lisbon
- Salam P. Bachour, Department of Neurology, University of Minnesota
- Uzma Samadani, Department of Neurological Surgery, University of Minnesota
- Geoffrey Ling, Department of Neurology, Uniformed Services University

TBI continues to be a major cause of death and disability around the world. Two million people suffer a TBI each year in the United States alone, and approximately 1 million of them require an emergency room visit; 500,000 are hospitalized, and 50,000 die. Recent wars in Iraq and Afghanistan, as well as the recent surge in civilian terrorism and suicide bombing attacks, have made blast-induced TBI (bTBI) an emerging civilian medical concern in the context of polytrauma. The etiology of bTBI is not well defined and may differ in many ways from penetrating TBI. Therefore, TBI in general and bTBI in particular pose a great clinical challenge to both military and civilian populations.

The cellular consequences of brain injury should be dealt with via approaches that enhance neuroprotection. Brain injury triggers cellular dysfunction and disruption of cell membrane homeostasis that leads to excitotoxicity, oxidative stress, and initiation of apoptotic cascades. A cascade of neurochemical activities induced by sudden interruption of normal physiological cerebral blood flow in response to stress signals at the cell membranes exacerbates neuronal injury. Reactive oxygen species (ROS) are involved with brain injury. During injury, mitochondria are the main intracellular source of ROS and are both responsible for oxidative stress and the victim of it. Mitochondrial dysfunction can persist for days after the initial insult, leading to neuronal cell death or apoptosis.

Therapeutic methods aimed at protecting and restoring mitochondria function should be considered an integral part of brain injury treatment. The published literature points to the need to develop mitochondrion-targeted interventions that can be applied to the acute stage to prevent ROS-induced injury and apoptosis as an adjunct to current clinical intervention. To address important gaps in the current knowledge of brain injury, the use of early antiapoptotic treatment of intravenous tauroursodeoxycholic acid (TUDCA) and sodium phenylbutyrate (SPB) administered after the onset of TBI and continued for the next three days post-injury should be examined. TUDCA can interrupt apoptosis by blocking classic mitochondrial death pathways while also significantly activating survival pathways. TUDCA is also believed to be able to reduce the symptoms of brain injury by modulating the neural stem cells pool. SPB is a small molecule that inhibits histone deacetylase activity and promotes the transcription of several genes, including that of DJ-1, one of the causative genes protecting mitochondria by ameliorating endoplasmic reticulum stress during brain injury.

We propose the use of a novel rat model of primary bTBI using a lithotripsy technique that has been recently developed in our laboratory to assess the therapeutic effect of TUDCA+SPB on TBI. The proposed insightful mechanistic studies will identify new therapeutic targets and are expected to result in the development of novel therapies for treatment of bTBI in a gender-specific fashion that can easily be translated to clinical research and can have a major impact on outcomes for patients with bTBI.

A Brief Review of Protective Engineering for Blast-Induced Human Injuries

Presenter: Joseph Hamilton, Karagozian & Case, Inc.

Additional authors:
- Joseph Magallanes, Joseph Abraham, Mark Weaver, and John Crawford, Karagozian & Case, Inc.

This presentation provides a brief review of protective engineering for blast-induced human injuries from the perspective of a small business performing research, testing, and design for

DoD and others for over 45 years. Most current engineering design criteria for scenarios involving blast effects rely on empirical data or engineering rules of thumb. Our experience with field testing has provided a good understanding of blast, impact, and shock loads and, to some extent, the risk of human injury. Due to the high expense and time-consuming nature of field testing, novel experimental methods are needed to generate a wider range of data. To this end, we have recently developed specialized laboratory-based methods to simulate blast, impact, and shock loads, which we will describe. Additionally, modeling and simulation can inform our understanding of phenomena governing neurological effects and threats, but this requires collaboration among multiple disciplines and very specialized inputs to validate, improve, and understand the implications of simulation results. We describe some of the most relevant considerations for modeling and simulation. We conclude with a survey of some recent protective designs that have the potential to mitigate risk of injury.

Bio-Templated Fluorescent Metal Nanocluster for Blast-Induced Injury Studies

Presenter: Shashi Karna, Army Research Laboratory, Weapons and Materials Research Directorate

Additional author:
- Raj K. Gupta, Department of Defense Blast Injury Research Program Coordinating Office, Army Medical Research and Materiel Command

Understanding the fundamental mechanisms of blast-induced injuries to human tissues has proved challenging despite extensive research efforts in recent years. Interaction of blast waves with the human system involves a complex set of linear and nonlinear phenomena with diverse chemical, mechanical, and biological effects. Among the parameters that play important roles are the local pressure, deposited energy, and onset of chemical and biochemical reactions. Currently, there are no reliable techniques to visualize and determine local pressure at the interaction site at the cellular level.

In an effort to address this issue, we have begun to create a nanoscale tool set that can be used to accurately image and establish local pressure experience by biological systems at the cellular level. The tool set consists of protein-templated metal nanoclusters that exhibit wavelength-tunable intense photoemission. The intensity of the fluorescence emission changes with local pressure and offers a powerful means of pressure detection for biological systems at the cellular level. This talk will present an overview of the chemistry, photo physics, and pressure responses of the fluorescent intensity in protein and tissue-templated metal nanoclusters.

PTSD-Related Behavioral Traits in a Rat Model of Blast-Related mTBI Are Reversed by the mGluR2/3 Receptor Antagonist BCI-838

Presenter: Georgina Perez-Garcia, Department of Neurology, Icahn School of Medicine at Mount Sinai, and NFL Neurological Care Center

Additional authors:
- Rita De Gasperi and Miguel A. Gama Sosa, Department of Psychiatry and Alzheimer's Disease Research Center, Icahn School of Medicine at Mount Sinai, and James J. Peters VA Medical Center

- Gissel M. Perez and Alena Otero-Pagan, James J. Peters VA Medical Center
- Anna Tschiffely, Richard M. McCarron, and Stephen T. Ahlers, Naval Medical Research Center
- Gregory A. Elder and Sam Gandy, Department of Neurology, Department of Psychiatry, and Alzheimer's Disease Research Center, Icahn School of Medicine at Mount Sinai

Blast-related mTBI is a frequent battlefield injury among soldiers deployed to the conflicts in Iraq and Afghanistan. In an animal model, Elder and colleagues previously showed that rats subjected to repetitive low-level blast exposure developed behavioral and cognitive abnormalities, including PTSD-related behavioral traits that were present many months after blast exposure.

TBI is reported to impair neurogenesis, raising the possibility that proneurogenic drugs might be effective in modifying the course of latent manifestations resulting from mTBI. Gandy and colleagues previously reported that pharmacological inhibition of mGluR2/3 receptors with BCI-838 leads to procognitive and anxiolytic/antidepressant effects in rodents (Kim et al., 2014). The aim of this study was to investigate whether administration of BCI-838 could enhance neurogenesis in the dentate gyrus (DG) of blast-exposed rats and reverse PTSD-related behaviors.

Methods: Two-month-old rats were subjected to three 75-kPa blasts under anesthesia. Beginning at two weeks post–final blast exposure, rats were treated daily with BCI-838 (4 or 10 mg/kg/day) for two months and tested on a variety of cognitive and anxiety-/stress-related behavioral tasks. Two weeks after beginning BCI-838 treatment, bromodeoxyuridine (BrdU) was administered intraperitoneally (150 mg/kg per day for one week), and effects on hippocampal neurogenesis were assessed.

Results: BCI-838 reversed anxiety in the light/dark emergence task and zero maze following blast exposure. BCI-838 treatment was associated with decreased fear memory in the cued fear conditioning test as compared to controls or to blast-exposed rats not treated with BCI-838. Moreover, four weeks after training, BCI-838 reversed the blast-associated impairment in recognition memory. Double immunolabeling with anti-BrdU and anti-doublecortin antibodies confirmed the proneurogenic effect of BCI-838 in the DG of drug-treated blast-exposed rats.

Conclusions: BCI-838 reversed PTSD-related traits in a rat model of mTBI, improving anxiety-related behaviors, fear memory, and long-term recognition memory. BCI-838 also increased neurogenesis in the DG of drug-treated blast-exposed rats. Current therapies are incompletely effective for treatment of PTSD-related symptoms following blast injury. The present study highlights BCI-838 and the mGluR2/3 pathway as potential leads to the development of novel pharmacological therapies for veterans suffering from PTSD symptoms following blast-related mTBI.

Funding: VA MERIT 1I01RX000684 (S. Gandy) and VA MERIT 1I01RX000996 (G. Elder).

Computational Mechanobiology of Neuronal Structures in Military Operational Repetitive Blast Exposures

Presenter: Andrzej J. Przekwas, CFD Research Corporation

Additional authors:

- Harsha T. Garimella and Mahadevabharath Somayaji, CFD Research Corporation
- X. Gary Tan, Naval Research Laboratory
- Reuben H. Kraft, Pennsylvania State University
- Raj K. Gupta, Army Medical Research and Materiel Command

bTBI has become a signature wound in the recent military operations and is becoming a significant factor of civilian blast explosion events. The increased awareness of the military and civilian neurotrauma has stimulated research in low-level repetitive blast and impact neurotrauma in military operational scenarios and civilian contact sports. Current understanding of bTBI mechanisms, particularly for low-level repetitive injury, is limited, and little is known about the short- and long-term sequela. Mathematical models of blast- and impact-induced TBI may provide a foundation to study these repetitive brain injury mechanisms and, perhaps, aid in accelerating the development of improved personal protective equipment and operational protocols, as well as neuroprotective and rehabilitation strategies. However, computational modeling of neurotrauma poses significant challenges, as it involves several physical and biomedical disciplines, as well as a range of spatial and temporal scales.

The majority of computational TBI research has focused on modeling macroscale brain tissue biomechanics and on head-scale brain injury criteria. Over the past few years, we have advocated and demonstrated the need for and benefits from the multiscale modeling of TBI. In this framework, the head/brain-scale injury biomechanics are coupled to the mechano-biology of neuronal structures, such as axons, synapses, cytoskeletal structures, and membranes. Multiscale models can also link the effects of "primary" microdamage to neuro-axonal structures with the "secondary" injury and repair mechanisms. However, the main challenges are to develop multiscale anatomical geometry models of the brain with "embedded" microstructures, to calculate loadings to these microstructures using macroscale results, and to "bridge" the acute primary injury to very-long-time-scale secondary injury and repair models.

This work introduces a novel multiscale simulation framework for bTBI based on CoBi tools with demonstrated models of both macroscale brain injury biomechanics and microscale mechano-biology models of synaptic, axonal, and cytoskeletal injury. Here, we present preliminary results of multiscale simulations of human body responses to low-level blast exposures during breacher and gunner training. The blast loads on the human head are used to simulate the macroscale human head/brain biomechanics, which are then transformed onto the "embedded" mesoscale axonal fibers present in the brain tissue.

We propose a novel framework for using the biomechanical response of these different axonal fibers to identify the areas of potential microdamage to neuronal structures and using this response for developing neuro-mechanobiology simulations of the evolution of microscale axonal and synaptic injury. These simulations demonstrate the structural changes to the synaptic clefts and postsynaptic densities and can be used as a starting point for modeling a cascade of secondary neurobiology effects, such as Tau phosphorylation and aggregation, disassembly of microtubule networks, blockage of intraaxonal transport, formation of axonal varicosities, beading, and retraction balls. A better understanding of the dynamics of diffuse synaptic injury may offer a window of opportunity in which an appropriate treatment may modify an imbalance between post-injury excitatory and inhibitory processes.

Transcranial Doppler Ultrasound as a Quantitative Biomarker in Evaluation of Mild, Moderate and Severe Traumatic Brain Injury: Current Status

Presenter: Alexander Razumovsky, Sentient NeuroCare/SpecialtyCare

This review paper summarizes the advantages of transcranial Doppler (TCD) ultrasound for patients with acute (moderate and severe) TBI to detect primary and secondary injury and guide therapy in patients to avoid cerebral ischemia due to the posttraumatic vasospasm and intracranial hypertension.

In critical care settings, multiple peer-reviewed publications show that TCD is predictive of angiographic posttraumatic vasospasm and onset of intracranial hypertension and is validated in numerous peer-reviewed publications. Moreover, in 2012 and 2015, DoD panels of experts determined that CT and TCD were the most useful modalities in the clinical setting for patients with moderate and severe TBI. The Army Medical Department TCD TBI program that started in October 2008 in several military hospitals also showed high clinical utility of TCD for acute moderate-to-severe war-time TBI patients. TCD clinical utilization as a quantitative biomarker and point-of-care ultrasound provides better detection, characterization, and monitoring of objective cerebral hemodynamics changes in symptomatic patients with combat-related TBI, including blast injuries. Finally, the brain's response to the long-term effect of mTBI is partially understood. The post-TBI status of cerebrovascular reactivity has important implications with regard to the treatment of long-term effects of mTBI. In addition, preliminary studies of active-duty service members many years after their last mTBI indicate that concussions lead to the vascular injury reflected in abnormally elevated cerebral blood flow velocities measured by TCD due to the enduring stenotic process and represent early signs of atherosclerosis. A paradigm shift in the importance of the vascular response to injury opens new avenues of drug-treatment strategies for mTBI.

TCD makes good clinical and economic sense, as it is a reliable, quantitative, and inexpensive "biomarker" for the acute clinical manifestations of moderate and severe TBI and the long-term effects of mTBI. TCD utilization will improve the sensitivity of neuroimaging of subtle brain perturbations, and combining these objective measures with careful clinical characterization of patients may facilitate better understanding of the neural bases and treatment of the signs and symptoms of TBI (mild, moderate, and severe).

The opinions and views expressed herein belong solely to the authors. They are not nor should they be implied as endorsed by the Department of Defense. This work was supported, in part, by the Army Medical Research and Materiel Command's Telemedicine and Advanced Technology Research Center, Fort Detrick, Maryland.

Exposure Standards Program: Neurological Correlates of Repeated Low-Level Blast Exposure in Career Breachers

Presenter: James Stone, University of Virginia

Additional authors:
- Stephen T. Ahlers, Naval Medical Research Center
- Nick Tustison, University of Virginia School of Medicine

Standards for repeated exposure to blast events do not exist. As the military considers deploying blast dosimeters operationally, there is a gap in knowledge to assess the risk of neurological effects associated with repeated "low-intensity" blast exposure(s). Occupational standards for acute exposure that guide safe distances and blast intensity are based on overt pathological outcomes and may not fully account for subtle neurological outcomes that are cumulative.

This is a programmed effort supported by investigators with extensive experience in the assessment of acute and chronic effects of blast exposure in military personnel and animal models. There are three program goals. The first major goal is to assess blast exposure effects in military operators by determining self-reported blast experience and symptoms, characterizing the biological response to blast exposure in the field, and assessing the cumulative effects of repetitive blast exposures over a career. The initial phase of this effort focused on breacher populations. One of the goals of the present effort is to explore neuroimaging correlates of repeated low-level blast exposure. The current study assessed 20 career breachers and compared them with 14 matched controls. Sequence acquisition occurred on a Siemens 3T system and included 3D T1-weighted sequences, DTI, and resting state blood oxygen level–dependent imaging to assess connectivity measures.

T1-weighted images were processed using the Advanced Normalization Tools (ANTs) cortical thickness pipeline. We employed a dimensionality reduction strategy for the structural analysis called eigenanatomy on both the ANTs-derived cortical thickness and log Jacobian maps. Eigenanatomy is a principal component analysis–based data decomposition technique with a spatial smoothness constraint that is used to determine the regions with the greatest variance. Regressing blast exposure on these eigen-regions showed a small effect ($p < 0.1$) in the cortical thickness maps and a larger effect ($p < 0.05$) in multiple eigen-regions of the log Jacobian maps. Regressing blast exposure on eigen-regions derived from axial diffusivity maps also demonstrated an effect ($p < 0.05$). Resting state functional MRI processing for the same cohort was performed using ANTsR (ANTs for R), which included motion correction, component-based correction, framewise displacement, and global signal nuisance regression. Power nodes were used to look at the relationship of functional connectivity in the default mode network to the level of blast exposure. Statistical significance was found in various connectivity measures (e.g., "centrality," "closeness"). In summary, initial analyses demonstrated differences in cortical, white matter, and connectivity measures in career breachers vs. controls. Analyses are ongoing related to the functional significance of these findings.

The Brain Gauge: A Neurosensory Assessment Tool That Reliably Tracks Brain Health

Presenter: Mark Tommerdahl, University of North Carolina

Additional authors:
- Eric Francisco and Jameson Holden, Cortical Metrics, LLC
- Oleg Favorov, University of North Carolina
- Laila Zai, Applied Research Associates, Inc.

A new system for assessing brain health that employs a portable computer peripheral (the Brain Gauge) to enable high-resolution tests of within-brain connectivity has been successfully developed. mTBIs are difficult to diagnose or assess and are particularly difficult to assess in circumstances where triage decisions are necessary. The majority of methods currently proposed to solve this problem are costly, nonportable, extremely slow, often invasive, and/or in many cases fail to definitively (and quantitatively) diagnose the condition or lack the resolution to assess treatment efficacy. Direct measures of brain health are difficult to achieve because of both the cytoarchitectural complexity of the brain and the resolution necessary to detect subtle changes in function.

The Brain Gauge system delivers tactile (skin) stimulation to the fingertips and leverages the neuroanatomical complexity that exists between the adjacent cortical areas that are activated by fingertip stimulation. The observed sensory percepts are highly influenced by interactions between adjacent brain areas and effectively provide a potentially high-resolution metric of functional connectivity. The protocols that were both designed and validated from in vivo studies of cerebral cortical dynamics in nonhuman primates target a number of information processing mechanisms and are called *cortical metrics*. These have been demonstrated in multiple independent studies to be sensitive to alterations in brain health.

The system has been reliably used in a diverse spectrum of neurological disorders (i.e., traumatic, developmental, degenerative, pharmacological) and has proved to be extremely sensitive to alterations in brain health. One of the strengths of the method is the correlation of the cortical metrics with measures obtained with an animal model, and the animal model allows for predictions of the impact of traumatic insult to the central nervous system. Viability of the method as an effective tool for tracking recovery from traumatic insult has been established in sports concussion studies (99-percent confidence level [$p < 0.01$]) for differentiating individuals with and without concussion. Studies in military populations have been initiated, and evaluation of subconcussive events is a new initiative. A major component of the current effort is the practical implementation of the method in the field, which includes delivery of easily interpretable results to end users. Observations obtained from both human and animal studies will be presented.

Appendix F. Expert Panel Biographies

A panel of subject-matter experts, including policymakers, clinicians, and scientists, helped lead and focus discussions during the plenary sessions. Expert panel members also chaired working group sessions in which participants addressed the four meeting questions.

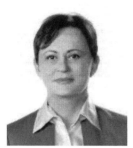

Ibolja Cernak

Dr. Cernak is president of STARR-C (Stress, Trauma and Resilience Research Consulting) LLC. She has broad multidisciplinary expertise, including an MD, an MS in biomedical engineering, an MS in homeland security (public health preparedness), and a PhD in pathophysiology and neuroscience. Previously, Dr. Cernak was a medical director and principal professional staff (tenured professor equivalent) at the Johns Hopkins University Applied Physics Laboratory; associate professor of neuroscience at Georgetown University, visiting professor at James Cook University in Townsville, Queensland, Australia; visiting professor at the 3rd Military Medical University, Chongqing, People's Republic of China; and professor of clinical pathophysiology in Belgrade, Serbia (formerly Yugoslavia).

With more than 30 years of experience, Dr. Cernak is world-renowned for her clinical and experimental research on blast injuries, including blast-induced neurotrauma.

Her research also includes traumatic brain injury of various etiologies focusing on the mechanisms of trauma-induced long-term neurological and mental health impairments, stress response and resilience to occupational stress, and predictors of injury and increased susceptibility to illnesses/injuries in military and first responder populations.

Dr. Cernak has published more than 200 research articles in international refereed journals, served as a keynote or invited speaker at more than 300 professional meetings, and filed three patents. She is a member of several professional bodies, including three subject committees of the Institute of Medicine, on the long-term consequences of traumatic brain injury in veterans, on soldiers' readjustment problems, and on the long-term consequences of blast exposure, as well as the NATO Human Force and Medicine task groups focusing on blast and other military injuries.

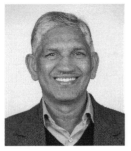

Namas Chandra

Dr. Namas Chandra is a distinguished professor of biomedical engineering and the founding director of the Center for Injury Biomechanics, Materials, and Medicine and the Institute for Brain and Neuroscience Research at the New Jersey Institute of Technology. He is also a fellow of the American Society of Mechanical Engineers and the American Institute for Medical Biological Engineering. Dr. Chandra has around 32 years of academic experience and nine years of industrial experience. He was a university distinguished research professor at Florida State University and associate dean for research at University of Nebraska, Lincoln. He has been continuously funded by DoD on studies of the micromechanics of materials and the biomechanics of blast-induced brain injury since 1987. His blast facility was recognized as a top 10 laboratory in the country by *Popular Science* and pioneered shock tube design. Dr. Chandra has published more than 225 articles, including 116 in archival journals, has been cited 4,160 times, has edited four books and two book chapters, and has presented at 75 colloquiums and six workshops. He has also supervised a total of 52 MS, PhD, and postdoctoral students. He was the chair of the expert panel for the 2014 SoSM meeting on environmental sensors.

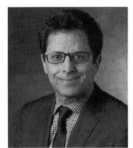

Jamshid Ghajar

Jamshid Ghajar, MD, PhD, FACS, is a clinical professor of neurosurgery and director of the Concussion and Brain Performance Center at Stanford University. He operates on acute, severe TBI at Stanford and directs the concussion clinics at the Stanford Neuroscience Health Center and at Stanford Sports Medicine.

He completed his MD/PhD at Cornell University Medical College, writing his PhD dissertation on neurochemistry and brain metabolism during coma. During his residency training at Cornell New York Presbyterian Hospital, he invented and patented several neurosurgical devices that are now used worldwide.

He is the founder and president of the Brain Trauma Foundation (BTF), which, since 1986, has worked with its partners to develop and maintain evidence-based guidelines on severe TBI. BTF's severe TBI guidelines are the standard of care for U.S. trauma centers and have led to a 45-percent decline in deaths.

Dr. Ghajar is the principal investigator for the DoD-funded Brain Trauma Evidence-based Consortium (B-TEC), a partnership between Stanford University, Oregon Health Sciences University, and other institutions. B-TEC and its partners maintain and update evidence-based guidelines for severe TBI and are charged with developing an evidence-based classification for concussion and TBI.

Dr. Ghajar founded SyncThink in 2009 to commercialize eye-tracking technology, useful in detecting visual attention impairments. He was the principal investigator on the DoD-funded EYE-TRAC Advance study to test 10,000 normal and concussed subjects using novel, portable eye-tracking goggle technology capable of assessing visual tracking impairments precisely and reliably within a minute. The technology received Food and Drug Administration approval in 2016. The SyncThink technology platform, EYE-SYNC, which uses Gear VR goggles with built-in eye trackers, has been adopted widely including, by all Pac-12 schools and the Golden State Warriors.

Jessica Gill

Dr. Gill is a tenure-track investigator at the National Institutes of Health and co-director of the biomarkers core for the Center for Neuroscience and Regenerative Medicine. Dr. Gill has an established clinical and laboratory infrastructure to examine the biological mechanisms of TBI and concussions and related comorbidities, including posttraumatic stress disorder, postconcussive disorder, depression, and neurological deficits.

Findings from her laboratory include alterations in tau and amyloid beta in acute and chronic TBI patients using an ultrasensitive laboratory method, and that tau elevations after concussions relate to a prolonged return to play. Dr. Gill also examines biomarkers of acute blast exposure, as well as biomarkers that relate to long-term symptoms and deficits. In addition, her studies link alterations in sleep regulatory proteins and the activity of genes that regulate sleep in patients with brain injuries. Other collaborations include analyses of genomic modifications in athletes and military veterans with repeated TBIs. The goal of Dr. Gill's laboratory is to determine the biological mechanisms of TBIs, blasts, and concussions and related symptoms in patients with repeated injuries, as well as the role of sleep in these biomarkers and patient outcomes.

James Zheng

Dr. James Zheng is director of the Technical Management Directorate and chief scientist for Project Manager Soldier Protection and Individual Equipment, Army Program Executive Office–Soldier.

Dr. Zheng has a bachelor's degree in chemistry and a master's degree in physics from the University of Science and Technology of China. He earned his PhD in physical chemistry from Purdue University. Dr. Zheng holds two patents and has published more than 70 scientific papers.

Dr. Zheng was one of the recipients of the Army's Greatest Invention Award in 2002 for developing a DoD standard body armor system, the Interceptor Multiple Threat Body Armor. He received the Army's Superior Civilian Service Medal in 2008 for "exceptional meritorious and superior technical achievement" for developing the Enhanced Small Arms Protective Insert. In 2009, he received the Program Manager of the Year award from Office of Secretary Defense Comparative Testing Office. He is one of the recipients of the 2013 Office of Secretary Defense Manufacturing Technology Achievement Award. In 2016, he received the Order of Saint Maurice medal from the National Infantry Association for "representing the highest standards of integrity, moral character, professional competence, and dedication to duty" and his second Superior Civilian Service Medal for "dedication to duty [that] has brought lifesaving personal protective equipment to hundreds of thousands of Infantry Soldiers and saved countless lives."

Appendix G. Meeting Participants

Yll Agimi
Defense and Veterans Brain Injury Center

Denes Agoston
Uniformed Services University

Stephen Ahlers
Naval Medical Research Center

William Ahroon
Army Aeromedical Research Laboratory

Regina Armstrong
Uniformed Services University, Department of Anatomy, Physiology and Genetics

Renee Attwells
Embassy of Australia

Monuel Aulov
New Jersey Institute of Technology

Ida Babakhanyan
Defense and Veterans Brain Injury Center

Amit Bagchi
Naval Research Laboratory

Jason Bailie
Defense and Veterans Brain Injury Center

Rohan Banton
Army Research Laboratory

Elizabeth Barrows
BarrowsMED

Jennifer Belding
Naval Health Research Center

Patrick Bellgowan
National Institutes of Health

Timothy Bentley
Office of Naval Research

Timothy M. Bonds
RAND Corporation

David Borkholder
BlackBox Biometrics, Inc.

Angela Boutte
Walter Reed Army Institute of Research

Patrick Brewick
Naval Research Laboratory

Kelley Brix
Defense Health Agency, Research and Development

Elizabeth Brokaw
MITRE Corporation

Catherine Carneal
Johns Hopkins University Applied Physics Laboratory

MAJ Walter Carr
Center for Military Psychiatry and Neuroscience, Walter Reed Army Institute of Research

Krista Caudle
Army Medical Materiel Development Activity

Ibolja Cernak
STARR-C (Stress, Trauma and Resilience Research Consulting) LLC

Steven Cersovksy
Army Public Health Center

Philemon Chan
L3 Applied Technologies

Namas Chandra
New Jersey Institute of Technology

David Cook
Department of Veterans Affairs, Puget Sound Health Care System, and University of Washington

A. Tamara Crowder
Office of the Assistant Secretary of Defense for Health Affairs, Health Readiness Policy and Oversight

Kenneth Curley
Army Medical Materiel Development Activity

Gregory Davenport
The Conafay Group

Thomas DeGraba
National Intrepid Center of Excellence, Walter Reed National Military Medical Center

Ramon Diaz-Arrastia
University of Pennsylvania

Ann Mae DiLeonardi
Army Research Laboratory

Jean-Philippe Dionne
Med-Eng, a division of the Safariland Group

CDR Josh Duckworth
Uniformed Services University

Lt Col Melinda Eaton
Army Medical Material Development Activity

Ashley Eidsmore
Army Research Laboratory

Greg Elder
James J. Peters VA Medical Center and Icahn School of Medicine at Mount Sinai

Kate Eltzroth
Martin-Blanck and Associates

Charles Engel
RAND Corporation

Katie Francia
Army Medical Research and Materiel Command, Joint Trauma Analysis and Prevention of Injury in Combat

Louis French
National Intrepid Center of Excellence, Walter Reed National Military Medical Center

MG Malcolm Frost
Commanding General, Center for Initial Military Training, Army Training and Doctrine Command

Elizabeth Fudge
Office of the Assistant Secretary of Defense for Health Affairs, Health Readiness Policy and Oversight

Eleuterio Galvez, Jr.
Army Medical Research and Materiel Command, Joint Trauma Analysis and Prevention of Injury in Combat

Jamshid Ghajar
Stanford University

Jessica Gill
National Institutes of Health

Raj Gupta
Army Medical Research and Materiel Command

Dallas Hack
Cohen Veterans Bioscience

Jonathan Hamilton
NPR News

Joseph Hamilton
Karagozian & Case, Inc.

Timothy Harrigan
Johns Hopkins University Applied Physics Laboratory

Katherine Helmick
Defense and Veterans Brain Injury Center

Lynn Henselman
DoD-VA Hearing Center of Excellence

CPT Bryan Henson
Office of the Commanding General, Center for Initial Military Training, Army Training and Doctrine Command

COL Sidney Hinds
DoD Blast Injury Research Program Coordinating Office

Emily Hoch
RAND Corporation

Michael Hoffman
Center for Devices and Radiological Health, Food and Drug Administration

Stuart Hoffman
Office of Research and Development, Department of Veterans Affairs

Christopher Hoppel
Army Research Laboratory

Cheryl Hull
Henry M. Jackson Foundation

Grace Hwang
Johns Hopkins University Applied Physics Laboratory

Erick Ishii
Department of Veterans Affairs

Todd Jaszewski
Combat Casualty Care Research Program

CAPT Thomas Johnson
Naval Medical Center, Camp Lejeune, North Carolina

Charles Jokel
Army Public Health Center, Deployment and Environmental Medicine

Antony Joseph
Naval Health Research Center and Illinois State University

Sharon Juliano
Uniformed Services University

Venkata Kakulavarapu
New Jersey Institute of Technology

Gary Kamimori
Walter Reed Army Institute of Research

Alaa Kamnaksh
Henry M. Jackson Foundation

Shashi Karna
Army Research Laboratory

Kacie Kelly
George W. Bush Institute, Military Service Initiative

Yeonho Kim
Center for Neuroscience and Regenerative Medicine, Uniformed Services University

Brian King
Georgia Tech Research Institute

Sindhu Kizhakke Madathil
Walter Reed Army Institute of Research

Michael Kleinberger
Army Research Laboratory

Timothy A. Kluchinsky, Jr.
Army Public Health Center, Health Hazard Assessment Program

Vassilis Koliatsos
Johns Hopkins University School of Medicine

Reuben Kraft
Pennsylvania State University

Theresa Lattimore
Army Office of the Surgeon General, Army Medical Command

Michael Leggieri
Army Medical Research and Materiel Command

Fabio Leonessa
Uniformed Services University

Kevin Lister
Corvid Technologies

Joseph Long
Walter Reed Army Institute of Research

LTC Thomas Longo
Army Training and Doctrine Command

Jia Lu
DSO National Laboratories

George Ludwig
Army Medical Research and Materiel Command

Aris Makris
Med-Eng, a division of the Safariland Group

Saafan Malik
Defense and Veterans Brain Injury Center

Donald Marion
Defense and Veterans Brain Injury Center

Robyn Matthews
Leidos

Crystal Maynard
Army Medical Research and Materiel Command

COL(R) Robert Mazzoli
DoD-VA Vision Center of Excellence

COL Dennis McGurk
Joint Program Committee–5, Army Medical Research and Materiel Command

LTC James McKnight
Army Medical Research and Materiel Command, Military Operational Medicine Research Program

Alessio Medda
Georgia Tech Research Institute

Natalya Merezhinskaya
DoD-VA Vision Center of Excellence

Catriona Miller
Air Force School of Aerospace Medicine

Seileen Mullen
Martin, Blanck and Associates

Ann Nakashima
Defence Research and Development Canada

John O'Donnell
Naval Research Laboratory

LT Uade Olaghere da Silva
Naval Health Research Center

Thomas O'Shaughnessy
Naval Research Laboratory

Anthony Pacifico
Congressionally Directed Medical Research Programs, Army Medical Research and Materiel Command

Michelle Padgett
Undersecretary of the Air Force

Assimina Pelegri
Rutgers University

Georgina Perez-Garcia
Icahn School of Medicine at Mount Sinai and NFL Neurological Care Center

Daniel Perl
Uniformed Services University

Elaine Peskind
Department of Veterans Affairs, Puget Sound Health Care System

Mathieu Philippens
TNO Defence Rijswijk (NLD)

Thuvan Piehler
Army Medical Research and Materiel Command

Marcello Pilia
Army Medical Research and Materiel Command, Combat Casualty Care

Ronald Poropatich
University of Pittsburgh

Leslie Prichep
BrainScope Company and New York University School of Medicine

Andrzej Przekwas
CFD Research Corporation

Raul Radovitzky
Massachusetts Institute of Technology

Murray Raskind
Department of Veterans Affairs, Puget Sound Health Care System

Terry Rauch
Office of the Assistant Secretary of Defense for Health Affairs, Health Readiness Policy and Oversight

Alexander Razumovsky
Sentient NeuroCare/SpecialtyCare

CDR Randy Reese
Naval Bureau of Medicine and Surgery

Jaques Reifman
Biotechnology High-Performance Computing Software Applications Institute and Army Medical Research and Materiel Command, Telemedicine and Advanced Technology Research Center

Shawn Rhind
Defence Research and Development Canada

Marten Risling
Karolinska Institutet

Tyler Rooks
Army Aeromedical Research Laboratory

Sujith Sajja
Walter Reed Army Institute of Research

Liming Salvino
Office of Naval Research

Chris Santee
Office of Naval Research

Robert Saunders
Naval Research Laboratory

Thomas Sawyer
Defence Research and Development Canada

Eric Schneider
University of Virginia

Sean Sebesta
Department of Defense/Department of the Army

Kristin Sereyko
RAND Corporation

Deborah Shear
Walter Reed Army Institute of Research

Richard Shoge
Army Medical Research and Materiel Command, Military Operational Medicine Research Program

Maciej Skotak
New Jersey Institute of Technology

Captain Jean-Christophe St-Maur
Canadian Special Operations Forces Command

James Stone
University of Virginia

Keith Stuessi
Defense and Veterans Brain Injury Center

Dwayne Taliaferro
Army Medical Research and Materiel Command, Congressionally Directed Medical Research Program

Terri Tanielian
RAND Corporation

David Tate
University of Missouri, St. Louis

Victoria Tepe
DoD-VA Hearing Center of Excellence

Mark Tommerdahl
University of North Carolina

Jonathan Touryan
Army Research Laboratory, Human Research and Engineering Directorate

Molly Townsend
New Jersey Institute of Technology

Laura Tucker
Uniformed Services University

Christy Ventura
Uniformed Services University and Henry M. Jackson Foundation

Bao-Han (Christie) Vu
Army Medical Research and Materiel Command, Congressionally Directed Medical Research Program

Tim Walilko
Applied Research Associates, Inc.

Julie Wilberding
Center for Neuroscience and Regenerative Medicine, Uniformed Services University

Mary Williams
Department of Defense Joint Non-Lethal Weapons Directorate, American Systems

Kurt Yankaskas
Office of Naval Research

Laila Zai
Lucent, LLC

James Zheng
Army Program Executive Office–Soldier

Mariusz Ziejewski
North Dakota State University

Appendix H. Previous State-of-the-Science Meetings

First State-of-the-Science Meeting, Non-Impact, Blast-Induced Mild Traumatic Brain Injury, Herndon, Va., May 12–14, 2009, https://blastinjuryresearch.amedd.army.mil/assets/docs/sos/meeting_proceedings/2009_SoS_Meeting_Proceedings.pdf

Second State-of-the-Science Meeting, Blast Injury Dosimetry, Chantilly, Va., June 8–10, 2010, https://blastinjuryresearch.amedd.army.mil/assets/docs/sos/meeting_proceedings/2010_SoS_Meeting_Proceedings.pdf

Third State-of-the-Science Meeting, Blast-Induced Tinnitus, Chantilly, Va., November 15–17, 2011, https://blastinjuryresearch.amedd.army.mil/assets/docs/sos/meeting_proceedings/2011_SoS_Meeting_Proceedings.pdf

Fourth State-of-the-Science Meeting, Biomedical Basis for Mild Traumatic Brain Injury Environmental Sensor Threshold Values, McLean, Va., November 4–6, 2014, https://blastinjuryresearch.amedd.army.mil/assets/docs/sos/meeting_proceedings/2014_SoS_Meeting_Proceedings.pdf

Fifth State-of-the-Science Meeting, Does Repeated Blast-Related Trauma Contribute to the Development of Chronic Traumatic Encephalopathy? McLean, Va., November 3–5, 2015, https://blastinjuryresearch.amedd.army.mil/assets/docs/sos/meeting_proceedings/2015_SoS_Meeting_Proceedings.pdf

Sixth State-of-the-Science Meeting, Minimizing the Impact of Wound Infections Following Blast-Related Injuries, Arlington, Va., November 29–December 1, 2016, https://blastinjuryresearch.amedd.army.mil/assets/docs/sos/meeting_proceedings/2016_SoS_Meeting_Proceedings.pdf

References

Belding, Jennifer N., "Occupational Risk Moderates the Relationship Between Major Blast Exposure and Traumatic Brain Injury," paper presented at the Seventh State-of-the-Science Meeting, The Neurological Effects of Repeat Exposure to Military Occupational Blast: Implications for Prevention and Health, Arlington, Va., March 13, 2018.

Carneal, Catherine, "An Enhanced Human Surrogate Head Model for Evaluating Blast Injury Mitigation Strategies," paper presented at the Seventh State-of-the-Science Meeting, The Neurological Effects of Repeat Exposure to Military Occupational Blast: Implications for Prevention and Health, Arlington, Va., March 13, 2018.

Cernak, Ibolja, "Impaired Stress Coping and Cognitive Function Caused by Blast Exposure," paper presented at the Seventh State-of-the-Science Meeting, The Neurological Effects of Repeat Exposure to Military Occupational Blast: Implications for Prevention and Health, Arlington, Va., March 13, 2018.

Dionne, Jean-Philippe, "Receiving a Multiple Peak Blast Dose in a Single Complex Blast Event," paper presented at the Seventh State-of-the-Science Meeting, The Neurological Effects of Repeat Exposure to Military Occupational Blast: Implications for Prevention and Health, Arlington, Va., March 12, 2018.

Duckworth, Josh, "Understanding Potential Neurological Consequences and Mechanisms of Repeated Blast Exposure," paper presented at Seventh State-of-the-Science Meeting, The Neurological Effects of Repeat Exposure to Military Occupational Blast: Implications for Prevention and Health, Arlington, Va., March 12, 2018.

Elder, Greg, "Blast-Induced 'PTSD': Evidence from an Animal Model," paper presented at the Seventh State-of-the-Science Meeting, The Neurological Effects of Repeat Exposure to Military Occupational Blast: Implications for Prevention and Health, Arlington, Va., March 13, 2018.

Institute of Medicine, *Gulf War and Health, Volume 9: Long-Term Effects of Blast Exposures*, Washington, D.C.: National Academies Press, 2014.

Kamimori, Gary, "Quantifying Occupational Blast Exposure During Military and Law Enforcement Training," paper presented at the Seventh State-of-the-Science Meeting, The Neurological Effects of Repeat Exposure to Military Occupational Blast: Implications for Prevention and Health, Arlington, Va., March 12, 2018.

Kim, S. H., J. W. Steele, S. W. Lee, G. D. Clemenson, T. A. Carter, R. Gadient, P. Wedel, C. Glabe, C. Barlow, M. E. Ehrlich, F. H. Gage, and S. Gandy, "Proneurogenic Group II mGluR Antagonist Improves Learning and Reduces Anxiety in Alzheimer Aß Oligomer Mouse," *Molecular Psychiatry*, Vol. 19, No. 11, November 2014, pp. 1235–1242.

O'Shaughnessy, Thomas, "Neuronal Response to Multiple Shock Tube Overpressure Exposures," paper presented at the Seventh State-of-the-Science Meeting, The Neurological Effects of Repeat Exposure to Military Occupational Blast: Implications for Prevention and Health, Arlington, Va., March 13, 2018.

Risling, Mårten, "Changes in Monoamine and Galanin Systems Following Single and Repeated Exposure to Primary Blast," paper presented at the Seventh State-of-the-Science Meeting, The Neurological Effects of Repeat Exposure to Military Occupational Blast: Implications for Prevention and Health, Arlington, Va., March 13, 2018.

Shanker, Thomas, and Richard A. Oppel, Jr., "War's Elite Tough Guys, Hesitant to Seek Healing," *New York Times*, June 5, 2014.

Teland, Jan Arild, *Review of Blast Injury Prediction Models*, Norwegian Defence Research Establishment, March 14, 2012. As of January 12, 2019: https://www.ffi.no/no/Rapporter/2012%20-%2000539.pdf

Walilko, Tim, "Predictive Injury Risk Curves for Blast-Related TBI Through Computational Modeling of Multi-Parametric Empirical Data," paper presented at the Seventh State-of-the-Science Meeting, The Neurological Effects of Repeat Exposure to Military Occupational Blast: Implications for Prevention and Health, Arlington, Va., March 13, 2018.